The Lion's Share

by
Roy Kumpe
written with
Jim Lester

Rose Publishing Co.
Little Rock, Arkansas

I don't know what your destiny will be, but the one thing I know—the only ones among you who will really be happy are those who will have sought and found how to serve.

Albert Schweitzer

Copies May Be Ordered From:
    Arkansas Enterprises for the Blind
    2811 Fair Park
    Little Rock, AR 72204

Remit $11.50 per copy.

ISBN No. 0-914546-45-7
Library of Congress Card Catalogue No. 83-61324

Published by Rose Publishing Co., Little Rock, Arkansas

Foreword

The tremendous growth and success of the Pre-Vocational Adjustment Center for the Adult Blind, adopted by the Lions Clubs of Arkansas in 1946, has been so extensive and far reaching during the past forty years that its beginning and history of services through the years should be recorded in book form for future reference.

The early success of this project initiated by the Lions of Arkansas soon attracted the support of the general public and Lions from other states in building, equipping and staffing the most widely known and accepted Vocational Rehabilitation Center for the Adult Blind in the world. This outstanding facility attracted trainees throughout the United States and many foreign countries who were financially supported by State Departments of Vocational Rehabilitation and governmental agencies.

This is a classic example of successful cooperation between the private sector and government agencies. From 1947 through 1982 more than 5,000 blind individuals received vocational training at the Center, representing 50 states and 53 countries. There isn't any possible way to measure the value of this activity in the hearts and minds of the individuals who were served at the Center.

This book is also a success story of a visually impaired person who learned at an early age that a great deal more can be accomplished by saying I must do something about that, rather than, something must be done.

Finis E. Davis
Vice President and General Manager
American Printing House for Blind
(1947-____)
President, Lions International
(1960-61)

iii

Contents

Preface

For over forty years I've been one of the luckiest men in the world. This good fortune has resulted from devoting my life to a single purpose—aiding blind people in restructuring their lives to become responsible and productive citizens. This cause has been my calling and my way of serving mankind. My career over these past four decades had paralleled a virtual revolution in the rehabilitation of blind adults and to have played a small part in these momentous changes has brought me considerable delight and satisfaction.

The present volume is therefore not an effort to tattle or reveal heretofore unpublished secrets about my colleagues, but rather to relate how things happened, tell some of the history of the rehabilitation movement and share a little of the joy that working to help the blind has brought me.

Except for recluses and hermits, life is a sharing of experiences and I have been blessed with the opportunity of knowing and working with a uniquely wonderful group of individuals over the span of my life. I would like to thank those people who have shared my life and made it such a rich experience—my family, my friends, business associates, members of Lions International, the members of the board of directors of the Arkansas Enterprises for the Blind, my colleagues both here and abroad who have devoted their lives to our cause and especially the thousands of courageous blind people who have built a new life for themselves. Most importantly, I would like to thank my wife Berenice for her untold hours of sacrifice and devotion.

CHAPTER 1

Ironton

Over the past forty years I have delivered hundreds and hundreds of after-dinner speeches to civic groups, community organizations and professional associations. Even with this experience, I knew the address I had to present the night of February 5, 1978 would be a unique, once in a lifetime opportunity. By the time my hands touched the familiar edges of the speaker's lectern, I felt sure everyone in the room could hear my heart thumping inside my chest. As the applause receded I took a deep breath and prepared to attempt to express my appreciation to the over 300 people who had attended the dinner in honor of my retirement.

The entire day had been an unforgettable series of events for me. David Pryor, the governor of Arkansas, had declared February 5 to be "Roy Kumpe Day" and friends and family from all over the nation had gathered at the banquet that evening at the Camelot Inn in Little Rock. That evening I found myself surrounded by representatives of the four pillars of my life—my family, my church, Lions International and political figures from throughout the state of Arkansas. During the dinner, I received a special award from the President of Lions International and the board of directors of the Arkansas Enterprises for the Blind, the organization I had founded and directed for over four decades, announced the establishment of a series of fellowships to be given in my name. I also received the "Executive Award" presented by the Greater Pittsburgh Guild for the Blind.

Following a beautiful invocation by my Pastor, Dr. Dan Kenner, and an illustrious group of speakers including Arkansas Governor David Pryor, Lions International President Joseph McLoughlin and former Lions International President Edward G. Barry, my turn came to respond to the

1

activities of that wonderful night. As I began to speak, I couldn't help but reflect on the journey that led me to that special evening. I thought of all the outstanding individuals with whom I had worked over the years, about some of the heartaches as well as the good times we had shared. I remember a host of victories and few defeats, and I contemplated the heroes and villians who had played key roles in my career. I thought of hows and whys and even a few ifs. Mostly, I pondered how thankful I felt to have been a part of a unique crusade—the movement to aid the blind adults of the world.

I couldn't help but recall the ignorance and the indifference I encountered early in my life when I tried to combat the myth that blind people are useless to themselves and to society. I thought of the skepticism that once greeted my assertions that individuals with visual handicaps could be productive citizens and not pitiful objects of charity. Fortunately during the last half century, I have witnessed the retreat of those attitudes and observed the dawning of a new era in the history of the blind.

My personal journey that led me to the podium that February night had been a long voyage, but not a lonely one. As I stood before the audience on my own special evening, I reflected on how the whole way had been filled with people, with excitement and perhaps most of all, with dreams.

My journey began on an overcast and frosty morning—January 18, 1910, when I was born in the back bedroom of a modest three-room house in the rural community of Ironton, Arkansas. Although I was the fourth child of Dave and Mary Kumpe, two daughters had died in infancy between myself and my older sister. Some years later after the addition of four more sisters and a brother, the Kumpe household was constantly alive with laughter and the sound of children at play.

We lived on a truck farm—about forty acres of woods and pastures where my father raised livestock and grew watermelon, cantaloupe and tomatoes. Back in those days my father had to get up at two o'clock every morning, load his produce on a wagon and travel twelve miles into Little Rock to the wholesale market where the grocers would gather to buy fruits and vegetables to stock their warehouses. From that situation I learned my first lesson in economics. As soon as the highways began to improve in the state, the farmers from south

2

Arkansas started hauling their tomatoes to Little Rock in trucks. Their tomatoes ripened a little earlier than ours and aided by improved transportation, they always got the top prices. By the time our local farmers' crop reached the market the prices had dropped. This circumstance served as a painful reminder to me that change is probably the only constant element in modern life.

Modernity was, in fact, not something that came quickly to Ironton. The people in Little Rock said we were 'way out in the sticks' and to some extent a pioneer atmosphere did characterize the place. I was a grown man before indoor toilets, electricity and automobiles made any inroads into the area. On the other hand, the community of my boyhood contained a strong element of unity and neighborliness—people caring about one another. Ironton had been settled by individuals who believed in hard work, sobriety and family, and their descendants tenaciously held to those values.

Above all else, religion permeated the community, and most of my earliest memories are closely tied with the little clapboard Baptist church of Ironton. Although my family existed somewhere below the poverty line as it would be defined today, we never thought of ourselves as poor, and the struggle with the mortgage, the droughts and the taxes never got so bad we didn't have a little something for the collection plate on Sunday morning.

The church had been established in 1892 by five residents of Ironton, four of whom were Kumpes. This support for the church continued and the year before I was born, my mother and father donated the land for the church's cemetery.

Although the preacher only came to Ironton twice a month, the church remained the social and recreational center of the community all during the week and I don't remember a prayer meeting, an ice cream social or a revival that the Kumpe family failed to attend. Two miles north of us there was a Methodist community and two miles south a small group of Campbellites or Disciples of Christ. I started teaching Sunday School at sixteen, but many years passed before I discovered exactly how those people's religion differed from ours and for a long time I thought my destiny lay in being a Baptist preacher who would save all those Methodists and Campbellites from

3

their evil ways and convert them to the true faith of the good Baptists of Ironton.

While our neighbors regarded my father as a leader in the church and in civic affairs, they recognized my mother as a worker. She worked in the home and she worked hard. She milked the cows, cared for the chickens, cleaned the house, did the laundry, tended the garden and if there was any time left she helped my dad in the fields. I recalled people saying my mother always "worked like she was fighting fire." But all that work left time for little else. Her formal education never went past the sixth grade and when we were growing up, she would always say, "I don't have time to read." Sometimes when she caught my father reading to us from newspapers or magazines, she scolded us and said we should quit wasting our time and get something done.

Like the rest of the Kumpes, Mother was a religious person, although I think she was a little shy about her religious feelings in front of other people. When we had prayer meetings or revivals, almost everyone would stand up and give testimony or witness, but my mother always remained quietly in her seat. I guess I was a little surprised when, later on in her life, after all the children had left home, my mother became active in several clubs and even began reading books. During those years she was able to turn her considerable energy into improving the school or the church grounds or organizing a pie supper or a social. When my mother died many years later, she left all of us a legacy of persistence and a respect for hard work. Even today, when someone asks me where I get my energy I often think of my mother attacking the endless chores of a farm wife with her unique brand of determination.

Another family trait that sprang from my early years in Ironton was fierce sense of independence. My father, who had only completed the seventh grade himself, always encouraged us to pursue the goals we wanted and not necessarily those someone else wanted for us. I remember one time a county extension agent came to our house and suggested my father consider sending my older sister Edna, to agricultural high school in Russellville. At that time many local farmers resented the county agents and often called them "smarty pants college boys" and accused them of meddling in "real" farmers' business. But Edna thought going to school was a wonderful idea and Dad said if that was the case, it was okay with him.

Unfortunately, the neighbors started gossiping about the matter and before too long, Edna's education became a community issue. Some of the local wags criticized Dad and kidded him by saying things like, "Dave, you're wasting your money. You don't need to educate girls. All they do in the end is get married and have kids. What do they need education for?" But my father's mind was set and all the teasing in the world was not going to change his decision. He found the money somewhere and sent my sister off to school, which turned out to be a pretty good decision. Edna became a teacher and later a family counselor and along the way provided a guiding light to the rest of us—encouraging and cajoling us to pursue our own educational goals, no matter what difficulties we faced.

My own sense of independence surfaced in a slightly different way. Although not demonstrative about her faith in public, my mother did have some definite ideas about religion in the home. For one thing, she refused to allow any playing cards in the house. In my mother's mind, cards inevitably led to gambling and other sinful activities. She regarded dancing in the same light. People who danced were liable to drink alchohol or fight or even worse, so dancing was also banned in the Kumpe household. However, when I was about sixteen, a family moved into the community from Little Rock. They had a Victrola and from time to time some of the younger people would stop by to listen to the records. One night a young lady from Sweet Home said she knew how to dance and put on a record and demonstrated the latest steps to the rest of us. This happened in the middle of the Roaring Twenties and I soon learned the steps and thoroughly enjoyed dancing whenever I could. Before too long word drifted out that some of the young people were getting together to dance and several of us anticipated a stern reaction in our own homes.

I knew my mother wouldn't like it but I didn't think my father would object. However, one night as I left the house, he stopped me and said, "Well, son, are you going out to dance again?"

"Yes sir," I said. "We probably will dance."

"Well, I'll tell you one thing," he said, taking a deep breath.

5

"I think you ought to make up your mind whether you are going to teach Sunday School or dance."

My father's comment left me stunned. I stood there for a long time and finally squared my shoulders and said, "Well, I believe I will keep on dancing."

Although I regarded my rebellion as rather minor, I think the Kumpes have always had an inclination toward an independent spirit. Take, for example, my great-grandfather, John Otto Kumpe. I first heard about him during World War I. In those days it was rather unpopular to have a German name or German ancestry. Even sauerkraut was called "Liberty Cabbage" back then. But my family had German heritage and we were certainly not ashamed of our background. Not that we weren't one hundred percent Americans. We were like most people—descendants of immigrants and proud of our family. As in most rural areas during the cold winter nights, the people in Ironton liked to gather around the stove or the fireplace and swap stories. By far the two most popular subjects were politics and religion. But once in a while, to my delight, somebody would tell the story of great-grandfather John Otto.

Born in 1807 in Hesse-Cassel, Germany, John Otto Kumpe early in life reflected a fiercely independent disposition. His widowed mother ran a jewelry store and had an older son who had served in the King's army. Fearing a similar fate for her younger son (many Hessian soldiers were hired out as mercenaries), she smuggled him out of the country and secured his passage on a ship bound for America. Although he was only nineteen years old at the time, he had completed a lengthy apprenticeship as a gardner with the Crown House of Hesse and when he arrived in the United States, he secured a job at the Botanical Gardens in Washington, D.C.

A few years later, John Otto migrated to Tuscumbia, Alabama, where he opened a bakery, purchased some land to farm and married a young lady from Tennessee named Lucinda Maples. By 1859 the couple had been blessed with twelve children and John Otto decided to move on again. They left Alabama in six wagons and made the long westward trek to Memphis, Tennessee. There, after selling the mules and the wagons, they loaded their belongings on a boat and traveled down the Mississippi to Arkansas Post and then up the Arkansas River to Little Rock.

6

Although Little Rock was a thriving frontier community, the town did not include a boarding house or even a hotel large enough to accommodate the whole family. John Otto then pitched a tent on the outskirts of town until he could rent a log cabin near a creek called the Town Branch. He proceeded to build a three-story brick building at the corner of Markham and Rock Streets, where the family lived upstairs while my great-grandfather operated a bakery and confectionery shop downstairs. Soon John Otto expanded his enterprise into the first toy store in the city and years later, when I was a boy, I met people who remembered that the most exciting event in the Christmases of their childhood had been a trip to Kumpe's store.

The Civil War, of course, wrecked Little Rock's economy, but in the postwar years John Otto began to expand his business holdings again. He purchased a considerable amount of local real estate, including a house at Fifth and Main where the Boyle Building is now located. Unfortunately, my great-grandfather's entrepreneurial skills did not include an ability to plan for the future. Unlike some of the other family businesses of the era like the Pfeifers or the Blasses or the Wortherns, John Otto Kumpe's holdings were not incorporated and when he died, the businesses and the properties were simply divided among his numerous heirs.

Part of my great-grandfather's property included farming acreage around Ironton. This was the land that eventually came to my grandfather, John Otto's oldest son, who also bore his name. Whenever people mentioned my grandfather's name around the stove or the fireplace their voices usually became hushed because no one ever knew quite what to make of the second John Otto Kumpe.

Along with three brothers, he served in the Confederate army, but somehow the second John Otto ran away, and whether from conviction or some other reason, wound up fighting in the Union army. Consequently, for a long time he was not welcome at home in Arkansas. After the war, he settled in the Smoky Mountain area of east Tennessee where he married a beautiful and somewhat mysterious girl named Oney Crutchfield. She had dark skin and straight black hair and some people said she was Portuguese. That observation turned out to be partially right. She belonged to the Melungeon

7

tribe, an unusual people created by frequent intermarriage between Portuguese sailors and Cherokee Indians.

Some years after his marriage, the younger John Otto became ill and wrote a letter informing the rest of the family that he needed their help. His father forgave him for his transgression during the war and I'm sure there was a tearful reunion when John Otto returned home. My great-grandfather quickly helped his son settle on some of the land at Ironton near several of his brothers. For a while the brothers operated a store and cotton gin to supplement the income from their farms. Tragically, the younger John Otto never fully recovered from an illness which he contracted during the war and died rather young. At the time, my father, the youngest of his children, was only two years old.

Some of the uncles helped raise the family and many years later my father used a small inheritance to purchase his own forty-acre tract in Ironton. Around that same time he met Mary Pritchard, the daughter of a sawmill owner in nearby Saline county, and after a proper courtship asked her to be his bride. That union produced a lifetime of happy memories and a few instances of genuine sorrow. Some of these later moments resulted from a set of circumstances that began to affect me in the spring of 1918.

As a child I had a normal share of misfortunes. At the age of four, I fell into a spring while trying to fill a bucket of water and almost drowned before my father could pull me out. About a year later, an old white mare we had on the farm got excited and kicked me in the head, which drew a lot of blood but did no serious damage.

Then, in my eighth year, something occurred that altered the course of my life. During the spring of 1918, a girl cousin from Wrightsville, Arkansas came to stay with our family for a while. Soon after she arrived she developed red, sore eyes which was not an uncommon ailment for rural children in those days. Since we all shared the same wash basin and the same towels, all the kids in our family and a good many neighborhood children came down with the disease. I remember my case being only slightly worse than the others. In fact, I thought I had almost recovered when I woke up one morning and discovered my left eye swollen shut. My mother tried salt water rinses and a few other home remedies, but

8

nothing seemed to have a lasting effect and about a month later I awoke and found the other eye in the same condition.

My parents took me to a country doctor, who prescribed more salt water rinses and for a while my sight improved. But throughout the summer, the sunlight irritated my eyes causing them to water and my vision to blur. That fall I started back to school for my third-grade year, but it soon became apparent that I could no longer read the blackboard. More ominously, the ailment worsened. Not only was my eyesight impaired but my eyes felt as if someone had thrown sand in them.

By this time my parents were extremely concerned and frightened. Obviously, I had something worse than red sore eyes. In desperation my father hitched up the wagon and took me to Little Rock to a doctor who sold eyeglasses. We bought a pair, but they were nothing but colored glass in a gold plated frame. My condition deteriorated and again my father hauled me to Little Rock for a visit with another physician. This doctor informed us that I had a disease called trachoma or granulated eyelids and needed an operation immediately.

I remember that first operation as the worst experience of my young life. The doctor turned the eyelid back and scraped away a series of tiny pimple-like growths on the inside of the lid. The unbearable pain made me think trachoma was surely the worst affliction known to man.

Trachoma is a virus infection with resulting vision impairment due to a scarring of the cornea. The disease originated in ancient Egypt and for a long time was referred to as "Egyptian Ophthalima." Around 1550 B.C. the standard prescription to combat trachoma included incantations and a solution of myrrh and cypress seeds applied to the eyes with a good quill—a treatment which was probably about as successful as the one I received from the surgeon in Little Rock.

In the nineteenth century, soldiers returning from faraway expeditions spread the disease. Both English and French troops who fought in Egypt in the early part of the century were stricken with trachoma and soon the malady reached epidemic proportions in England and France. Although a few cases occurred in colonial America, the disease only became widespread in the mid-nineteenth century in the

United States when an influx of immigrants carrying trachoma arrived from Europe. By 1897, however, the American government prohibited immigrants showing signs of trachoma from entering the country.

In the United States the disease became predominant in the mountainous areas of Tennessee, Kentucky, West Virginia and the Ozark regions of Missouri and Arkansas. Oddly, while black Americans appear to be immune to trachoma, American Indians are particularly susceptible to the virus.

Long after I suffered from the first attack of granulated eyelids, medical science brought trachoma under control though the use of sulfa drugs and by midcentury the disease had been virtually eliminated as a cause of blindness in the United States.

But in 1918 trachoma was a real and terrifying experience. After the first operation, my father found it increasingly difficult to take me to Little Rock several times a week for treatment. He simply could not spare the time away from the farm. The doctor helped solve the problem by suggesting that my father enroll me as a student in the state School for the Blind in the city. This idea seemed like a good plan since he served as the doctor for the school and could perform any additional surgical procedures at the infirmary on the campus. My mother said little about the matter. She wanted me to stay home, but there were other children to care for and she knew the travel put a strain on my father. So together my parents made the decision to enroll me.

Located at Eighteenth and Center Streets, the Arkansas School for the Blind dated back to the 1850s and the efforts of a blind Baptist minister in Arkadelphia to bring some rudimentary education to blind children. During the next decade, Otis Patton, the first superintendent, managed to secure a small appropriation from the state legislature and then in 1868 the school moved to Little Rock. The day my father left me at the institution my knees trembled and my lower lip quivered all morning. But I never cried. I guess I thought that made me a big boy.

By the time I arrived that fall, school had already been in session for a couple of weeks, which put me at a considerable disadvantage. Being the new student—the outsider—my classmates did not hesitate to inform me of my lowly status. I could see more than most of the children and I saw a terrifying group of blind strangers, some with grotesque deformities all of them going out of their way to reject me. Never in all the years since that day have I felt such a deep sense of loneliness and isolation.

Before I could begin to make friends, my problems actually increased. One of the worst flu epidemics in the state's history struck Little Rock that fall and about two weeks after I arrived at the School I began running a fever. On Saturday, the school nurse told me I would have to go to the infirmary — information I regarded as the most disastrous news imaginable. I suffered from an inordinate fear of hospitals and in my confused eight-year-old mind a hospital was where a person went to die. I pleaded with the nurse not to send me. Since my father planned a visit that day, I begged her to at least wait until he arrived and she reluctantly yielded.

The instant my father walked through the door, I abandoned all hope of being a big boy and dissolved into tears. I finally managed to explain to him about the nurse's fiendish plot and told him in no uncertain terms that I wanted to go home. He had already spoken with the doctor and knew I would be properly cared for in the school infirmary, but convincing me was another matter. He promised to take me into town for a soda or some candy while we discussed the situation. I agreed to that idea but before we left an unusual turn of events occurred.

As a courtesy, my father stopped at the superintendent's office to inform the proper authority that he was taking me off the campus for a while. This should have been a routine matter, except for some reason the superintendent became extremely hostile and informed my father that he couldn't take me away from the school under any circumstances. My father, who was a genuine individualist in his own way, shook his head and replied, "He is *my* son and I can do anything I want with him."

"Well, if you take him off the school grounds," the superintendent snapped, "you can't bring him back."

"Okay, son." My father turned to me. "Let's go pack your things. It's a long way back to Ironton."

I remember being ecstatic as I crawled into my own bed at home that evening. Even a serious case of the flu failed to spoil

11

my homecoming. But because of a high temperature I spent a restless night dreaming about blind boys. Big blind boys. One of the largest boys had a cane chair on his head (they repaired chairs at the school) and he began chasing me. Only I couldn't see where to run. I couldn't get away. Then the other blind boys began pursuing me waving their arms in front of them. I woke up screaming.

I stayed in bed for a week and although physically I felt awful, I experienced tremendous relief when I realized my father had no intention of sending me back to the school for the blind. Before Christmas I underwent another painful scraping operation on my eyes but I remember being extremely thankful to spend the holidays at home with my family.

Early in January, 1919, the governor fired the superintendent of the Arkansas School for the Blind amidst rumors of mismanaged funds and drug use. Colonel George Thornburg, a Little Rock attorney and prominent Mason, received the appointment as the new superintendent. Despite the fact the colonel had no formal qualifications as an educator or any background in working for the blind, he was an honest man who believed in the school's mission.

Later that same month my father received a letter from Colonel Thornburg apologizing for the ugly incident with the old superintendent and asking my father to reconsider enrolling me in the school. By this time I had reluctantly come to the same conclusion. If I remained at home I knew I would always be treated like an invalid. Long after I had recuperated from the flu, my parents kept me in bed as much as possible. They found it easier to wait on me than to have me stumbling around the house. While my mother and father believed that was the best way to care for me, I felt a terrible sense of helplessness and frustration to a degree that the memory of that experience profoundly influenced some important decisions later in my life.

In February, I returned to Little Rock where the new superintendent placed me in the third-grade class. Although I felt glad to be back in school, I soon discovered that acquiring an education was not going to be an easy task. The first thing I needed to know was how to read braille: the system of raised dots that enables the blind to "see" with their fingers. To this end, the teacher at the school handed me a thick braille book and said, "You'd better learn this quickly because you're already behind the other children." Then she walked away. No instructions. Just a book full of unfamiliar prickly dots. I found out later that the teacher was actually the wife of the school purchasing agent and could not read braille herself. At that time many of the teachers had only eighth-grade certificates and hardly any of them had had training to work with the blind. The memory of this lack of professionalism became another factor that years later played an important role in my life. But back then my major concern centered on conquering the mysteries of braille.

The concept of reading by raised dots originated with Charles Barbier, a French Signal Corps officer, who developed a system of "night writing" to enable his men to send coded messages at night. In 1820, Barbier presented his system to the Paris School for the Blind, where, although a clumsy process, its potential was recognized by a brilliant blind student named Louis Braille. Braille refined the method, cut the number of dots in half and developed the system that now bears his name. I finally learned to read Braille's dots by asking my fellow students for help. Despite my earlier conflict with some of the boys in the school, a few of them were kind enough to demonstrate how the pattern of dots worked and slowly the world of reading by touch opened to me.

During that time I always regarded my stay at the Arkansas School for the Blind as a temporary one. My eyes seemed to be improving and I firmly believed that before too long I would be back in public school. In fact, every doctor I visited held out that hope.

But in the summertime my condition always deteriorated. I simply could not bear the sunlight and eventually I spent my daylight hours in a room with windows covered by a thick quilt. I could go outside after dark, but even the dim glow of a full moon hurt my eyes.

Before I reached adolescence, I underwent several additional operations. Back then physicians used ether or chloroform as an anesthetic and each time I went under I thought I would die and never see my family again. I finally convinced the doctor to utilize a local anesthetic so I could stay awake even through the unbearable pain. But despite all the surgery, the cure proved worse than the disease. The scraping and burning of the lids created a residue of scar tissue on the cornea which ultimately caused permanent impairment of my sight.

I spent my twelfth summer in a special trachoma hospital run by the U.S. Public Health Service in Russellville, Arkansas. I liked the place because it never seemed like a hospital. We lived in an old rambling Victorian house with a huge lawn and, since the staff never gave us much to do, the patients played croquet in the back yard. Almost sixty years later I still enjoy playing croquet — a marvelous game for all ages.

That same summer I received my first sex education. Among the older blind fellows at the Russellville institution sex seemed to occupy every minute of conversation. We relaxed on the porch in the evening and all those men ever talked about were their sexual exploits, both real and imagined. Although I could not always distinguish the two, I still considered those evenings an important addition to my general knowledge of the world.

Later in the summer I met a man from New Mexico who was obsessed with going to Los Angeles for a series of chiropractic adjustments. He had done this once before and claimed that after those treatments he didn't have to undergo any more painful eye surgery and his vision had cleared to the point that he had been able to resume his job as a section foreman on the railroad. His story fascinated me. Since I had already suffered through seven hideous scraping operations, the hope of improved vision without surgery sounded like a miracle. My spirits soared when the man told me he thought the chiropractor could particularly help me since I had developed something of an abnormal posture by hanging my head to protect my eyes from the light.

I begged my father to allow me to visit a chiropractor. At first he thought I meant some kind of faith healer and refused to let me go. Fortunately my sister Edna intervened, explained the situation to our father and even offered to escort me to the chiropractic clinic. Finally my father relented and gave his approval.

I made an appointment with a chiropractor named Dr. Amy Barnett. She immediately started me on a series of adjustments and altered my diet, putting a heavy stress on vegetables and decreasing my meat consumption. After a while I began walking erect again and my eyes began to tolerate more light. The following summer I found I could even do some work around the farm and when I returned to school I no longer had to undergo the painful treatments in the hospital. Instead, I visited Dr. Barnett two or three times a week.

I recognized that chiropractic science is a controversial area and do not pretend to have thoroughly researched the entire matter. However, my own experience with chiropractors has been a beneficial one and to this day I am still a chiropractic enthusiast. My early experience with Dr. Barnett relieved a lot of my suffering and freed me from the agony of having my eyelids burned and scraped and for that I shall be eternally grateful.

Following my summer in Russellville I settled down to completing my education at the School for the Blind. Along with the regular academic curriculum, the school offered a variety of vocational programs, but I found none of them to my liking. For example, the school put considerable emphasis on music. One of the myths surrounding blind people is that because they are blind they have an instinctive ear for music and are "natural" musicians. The school staff believed that even if you could not be a professional musician, you could at least tune pianos for a living. Not in my case. The notes all sounded pretty much the same to me. Some were louder than others and occasionally I could tell one was higher or lower than another one. But not always. I simply had no talent for music and my music teacher finally suggested I seek other vocational interests—advice with which I agreed wholeheartedly.

I had better luck with broom making. Thanks to manual dexterity, I became one of the better students in the broom-making shop. One summer the instructor asked me to stay at the school and help him make brooms for other state institutions. I remember he said he could pay twenty-five cents an hour plus meals, which I thought constituted a marvelous wage. I had a similar experience with chair caning. Another student and I got quite a bit of chair work and were always able to make a little pocket money. By the time I turned fourteen, I made enough money in the chair and broom business to buy all of my own clothes and have ample spending money left over.

15

During my student days chair caning, broom making and piano tuning constituted the traditional vocational pursuits of graduates of the School for the Blind. Although I became skilled in two of these areas, I never seriously considered spending the remainder of my life engaged in either one. I had other ambitions. I wanted to go to college and then study law. Unfortunately, I heard few encouraging words in the pursuit of these aspirations. In my senior year most of my teachers tried to gently dissuade me from going to college. They all wanted to save me from a terrible disappointment. They explained that while I had the mind to achieve my goals, I might not be able to overcome my visual handicap — by that time I was regarded as legally blind.

Legal blindness is an often misunderstood term and is not the same thing as total blindness. Legal blindness is rather a deep twilight land of partial sight. Technically, the term means 20/200 in the better eye after the best correction, or the ability to see something at twenty feet that people with 20/20 vision can see at two hundred feet. Actually, only a relatively small percentage of blind people have no light perception at all. A common misconception is that if you can perceive light you are not really blind. As a young man, I could see much better than I can now, except for those summers many years ago when the light particularly irritated my eyes. Even during the best of times I remained visually handicapped, which many people around me felt would be an unconquerable barrier in trying to accomplish the goals I had set for myself.

Numerous polls and studies have revealed that, second to cancer, most people regard blindness as the most frightening affliction of all. In my own case, at first I had an irresistible tendency to ask, "Why has this happened to me?" In searching for the answer to that question I quickly concluded it was not only an unanswerable inquiry but that it was counterproductive even to ask. The question itself leads to self-pity and that never accomplished anything. What happened to me was something that simply happened — a throw of dice. The important thing was to look ahead — to set my goals high and find the way to achieve those goals.

I felt I had taken the first step toward my personal objectives when I graduated as valedictorian from the Arkansas School for the Blind in 1929. For my commencement address I selected the theme of service to my fellow man, which I regarded as an important long-range goal. My short-range plans still included college and law school and I felt more determined than ever that my visual handicap would not stop me. I knew the mountain might be treacherously high, but I was eager to begin the climb.

CHAPTER 2
Dreams and Realities

During the 1930's, the era of the Great Depression, the American people underwent a frightening interlude of uncertainty and anxiety. In many ways my own life at that time paralleled the strange odyssey of the nation as a whole. As the Roaring Twenties faded into history, I found myself trapped in a set of discouraging circumstances, my personal goals temporarily thwarted. But again, like the experience of the nation, out of that period of disappointment came a time of great hope and a renewed sense of purpose in my life.

Between the great crash of 1929 and the bombing of Pearl Harbor, I struggled through my education, both in school and in the world at large. I met and married the girl of my dreams and I discovered my life's work. The decade was a season of growth during which I built the foundations for exciting years that followed. By the close of that era I had accomplished some of the dreams of my childhood, while others had been tempered by reality.

My first dream centered on a college education. Originally I had hoped to attend the University of Arkansas, but because I feared finding "readers" in Fayetteville would be difficult, I chose Little Rock Junior College instead. LRJC proved to be an excellent selection since the change from the School for the Blind left me in a temporary state of confusion. In high school we only had three or four students in each class while college classes ranged from twenty-five to thirty people. I could not read the blackboard and even though I could write some because I had gone though the third grade in public school and understood the theory of writing, my abilities were inadequate for college work. The School for the Blind never required written work and it took a lot of practice to be able to write as well as my classmates at LRJC.

18

Another shock involved the amount of reading required. Since I could not afford a formal reader, my father and my younger sister Zelma read all my lessons aloud in the evenings. Even with their help, I sometimes felt I would never complete the necessary assignments in courses like history and literature. An important skill I did cultivate from that experience involved training my mind to outline material as it was being read and then seize the important points. Years later I found this aptitude to be one of the most valuable faculties I developed in school.

Although the time needed for my academic work combined with hitchhiking eight miles between Ironton and the campus limited my extracurricular activities, I tried to make the most of the opportunities I had. People with visual handicaps often work extra hard to prove they can do what other people are doing and I was no exception. I joined several service and social clubs and although I couldn't participate in football or basketball, I did make the track team, anchoring the mile relay and running the quarter mile. I remember one of my happiest moments in college occurred during a dual track meet with Monticello A & M. Their relay team was far ahead by the time I received the baton for the last lap and since I couldn't see how far behind I was, I started running as hard as I could. Having spent what felt like my last ounce of energy, I caught the A & M anchor man a few yards from the finish line and surged past him to win. I have always regarded that race as one of the more symbolic events of my youth.

I liked to compete and as a result, my biggest disappointment in college came when the faculty denied me the opportunity to participate on the debating team. Since I intended to become a lawyer, I knew how important debating could be for my future. The instructors who coached the team, however, had other ideas. They told me that even though I qualified for the team, they did not think it would be a good plan for me to debate because the time involved might harm my other studies. I regarded the whole experience as a severe blow, but one that seemed typical—being visually handicapped and having well-meaning people decide what is good for you instead of allowing you to decide for yourself. I remember I did receive some gratification when a young girl who made the team came to me one afternoon and confessed she did not know

19

anything about debating and asked me to coach her. I agreed and much to my satisfaction, by the end of the year she became one of the best debaters on the squad.

I had another unsettling experience in school, but this one did not surprise me at all. An instructor at the college took a personal interest in me and when he found out about my plans regarding the law, he arranged an appointment for me with a prominent downtown attorney named Graham Hall. When I went to see Hall he immediately began to point out all the problems a visually handicapped person would have in trying to study law. He droned on and on until finally eyesight seemed to be the only requirement necessary to become an attorney. I know he meant well, but I didn't relish the discouragement.

In October of my first year at Little Rock Junior College the stock market collapsed and pervasive clouds of gloom began to settle over America. The following summer, Arkansas experienced a terrible drought that ushered in the Great Depression. What that era meant in personal terms was there would be no money for education. No more LRJC. My family took a fatalistic view, saying, "Come on home, Roy, and we will all starve together." Only I wasn't about to starve. I had dreams. I was still going to become a lawyer. But I did realize that for the time being, my dreams would have to take a back seat to some harsh realities.

During my last year at the School for the Blind, a salesman passed through Ironton selling bibles to earn money to go to college. My father invited him to spend the night with us and the younger man convinced me I too could become a bible sales- man. As a result of that one conversation the next summer I hitchhiked to Nashville, Tennessee to take a week-long course in salesmanship from a company called Southwestern Book Publishers. After the lessons I journeyed to Charleston, South Carolina to begin my career as a door-to-door bible salesman. The whole summer provided me with a cornucopia of life experiences. For example, the school taught us never to argue with anyone. If the lady of the house told you black was white, you did not have to agree with her, you just said, "Come to think of it, black is a peculiar color." Since bibles were my business, oftentimes people would want to discuss religion and I found this to be a broadening expansion of my education. Being a staunch Baptist from rural Arkansas, I had no idea there was such a variety of religious interpretations: Methodist, Presbyterian, Jehovah's Witness, Catholic, Jewish. That summer I began a lifelong interest in the nature of religion and comparative faiths.

The summer of 1929 I traveled the back country of South Carolina with a sample case of Family Bibles, Teachers' Bibles, Enlargement Bibles and other religious books. The system required that we leave headquarters on Monday morning and not return until Saturday afternoon. We were on our own to live on whatever we collected and on the hospitality of the good people of South Carolina. Around four o'clock each afternoon, I would begin to look for someone in the neighborhood who might be willing to put me up for the night. Usually, I would sell that person a bible and then deduct a small credit for lodging.

Selling was a rigorous life and many of my fellow bible salesmen became homesick and quit. Once I even recruited four or five of my friends from the School for the Blind, but they all lacked the determination to see the project through. On several occasions I had to "postpone" a meal until I could make another sale because my pockets were empty. I also suffered continuing problems with my sight. The summer sun irritated my eyes and I never knew when I might wake up and find them swollen shut. I had to memorize the prospectus in order to demonstrate to the customers how to use the bible as a reference source and hide the fact I couldn't read the material. In retrospect, this situation seems ironic, because today we train people to accept their handicap and not try to conceal it.

The company challenged us to sell on holidays and I remember working on the Fourth of July because our supervisor told us we could celebrate Independence Day by being independent enough to get out and work. But the second summer I sold bibles, independence was not enough. The ravages of the Depression hit rural South Carolina with colossal force and few people had enough money to purchase a new bible. Even those who signed up to buy one at the beginning of the summer had no money to pay me when I made my deliveries in August.

When I realized there would not be sufficient money to return to college in the fall of 1930, I set out to earn enough funds to finance my education the following year. Since selling books could not produce the needed income, I secured a position with an insurance company. I sold a variety of small policies and had to go back to the policy holders and collect five cents every week — a lot of work for a minuscule return. I moved on to selling magazines door-to-door on a commission basis with a group called the Woman's Home Companion Reading Club. We sold magazine combinations and rotated work crews between Little Rock, Ft. Smith, Texarkana and Shreveport. I had a little more success at this job and when the company offered me a higher paying position in Jackson, Mississippi, I headed for the Magnolia State. While living in Jackson, I flirted with the idea of attending law school there and perhaps getting involved in Mississippi politics. I quickly discovered this plan would never be more than a dream since Mississippi politicians were born, not bred. Several friends politely informed me that if you did not come from the "right" families in the state, you would always be considered an outsider.

After a while, the magazine business dried up and I drifted back to selling bibles, this time in the coal mining areas of West Virginia. One year quickly turned into two and the two stretched into three. Each year I would think surely next year I will make it back into school, but as time went on my disappointment became critical. Still determined to be a lawyer, I felt the sting of inaction, unable to move toward my life's goal. In those days, if you married, that ended any hope of education because you had to work to support your wife and family. So I vowed I would not think about marriage until I had my law degree, and again I felt paralyzed. The years between 1930 and 1936 were disillusioning and frustrating ones; all of my dreams deferred. But somewhere deep inside of me I knew those dreams would someday become realities.

I decided to become a lawyer around the age of twelve. Back then my father served as the Justice of the Peace in Ironton, and since he had some political influence with the people in the community, politicians always called on him and visited our house. I also attended numerous political rallies in those days and I observed that many important political figures into a political career.

By the time I turned sixteen I had found a hero and role model in a young gubernatorial candidate named Brooks

22

Hays. Not only an attorney and prominent politician, Hays was also an active Baptist layman; a dynamic combination in the eyes of a young country boy. In 1926, I supported Hays' candidacy for governor despite the fact that my father actively campaigned for his opponent, Harvey Parnell. I made my maiden political speech on Hays' behalf and although I'm not sure how many votes my speech swayed, I know over the summer I talked one person into voting my way. That was the first year my mother qualified to vote by paying a poll tax and after much discussion I convinced her to vote for Brooks Hays. My father always laughed about the split in the family and good naturedly threatened to never pay another poll tax for my mother since she wouldn't support his candidate.

At that time I still hoped my sight would somehow return to normal and I would pursue the same path as Brooks Hays. By 1936 I had become more realistic about my handicap, but just as determined to pursue my career. During a visit to Little Rock I ran into an old classmate from my junior college days who attended the night law school in the city. He was enthusiastic about his studies and the school sounded like a wonderful opportunity. After several sleepless nights, I decided to compromise on my dream of having another full year of college and enrolled in that same night law school.

Since I needed financial assistance to continue my education, I talked to the superintendent at the School for the Blind about the possibilities of a stipend to hire a reader. I even got my father to come to the courthouse in Little Rock and inquire about special assistance for tuition or books, but he also found that nothing was available.

I remembered a couple of crippled students at junior college who I knew had received financial aid from the state, so I pursued the matter. What I discovered shocked me. Under the existing vocational rehabilitation law, blind people were considered non-feasible. The state could spend money for vocational training, but this meant short-term training like assisting a man who lost a leg to learn to be a bookkeeper or a cobbler. The rehabilitation people informed me that they considered the blind "non-feasible" because the cost of aiding them would exhaust most of the department's annual appropriation.

Eventually I secured an appointment with Ashley Ross, the head of vocational rehabilitation. He was a kind gentleman and finally agreed that under the circumstances the state could provide half of my law school tuition. The next year, since my grades were good, Mr. Ross expanded my aid to include the cost of my books and all of my tuition. Although I sold cemetery lots and clerked at J.C. Penney Store to pay for my room and board in town I was extremely grateful for the state aid. I could not have completed my studies without Mr. Ross' help and my dream of becoming a lawyer would never have come true.

When I finished law school in 1938, the economic problems of the Depression had still not been solved and rather than hang out my shingle as a fledgling attorney, I accepted a temporary position with the Rural Electrification Administration. I had earlier served on a committee to secure electrical service for Ironton and regarded my new position an expansion of that work. In coordination with the county extension office, I canvassed a four-county area to extend the services of the First Electric Cooperative of Jacksonville.

In the course of my job, I became acquainted with an elderly gentleman who lunched at a boarding house near our headquarters. One day the man approached me about representing a friend of his who, during a recent illness had made arrangements with a woman neighbor to care for him. In return he had deeded her a forty-acre tract of land. She had reneged on her part of the bargain and when the man regained his health I had my first law case. By recovering the client's property I received a $250 fee, which was quite a handsome sum in those days, and I hoped the case would be the beginning of a long and distinguished legal career. But while the law had opened doors for other opportunities and held the hope of a promising future, along the way I had developed some new interests.

My own experiences had led me to realize how much discrimination visually handicapped people suffered in terms of education, rehabilitation and employment opportunities. My valedictory speech at the School for the Blind had been on the theme of service and I wanted to channel some of that service into helping the blind. Although I didn't realize its significance at the time, an event had occurred in 1936 that

24

ultimately gave me an opportunity to implement that service and in turn altered the course of my life.

In that year the Congress of the United States enacted the Randolph-Sheppard Act. This legislation provided for the establishment of vending stands to be operated by blind individuals in federal buildings througout the country. The stands would sell newspapers, magazines, candy and tobacco products and would be licensed by the state agencies for the blind. Hailed as a major breakthrough in vocational opportunities for the visually handicapped, the Randolph-Sheppard Act supplied the chance for thousands of blind persons to become self-supporting and demonstrate they could be competent, contributing members of the American work force.

Guy Smith, a blind chiropractic doctor and the President of the Arkansas School for the Blind Alumni Association, first alerted me to the act after he read an article on the subject in the *Matilda Ziegler Magazine For The Blind.* Since I chaired the alumni's legislative committee, I began to follow the progress of the bill and study the background of the legislation. The history of the act dated back to the early 1920s when blind persons began operating lunch counters in industrial plants in Ohio, Michigan and some New England states. Most of these enterprises failed because of poor equipment and limited stock. A similar and more successful effort emerged at approximately the same time in New York City where a municipal ordinance granted World War I veterans with service-connected disabilities preference in acquiring newstand locations throughout the city.

These pioneering ventures stimulated the imaginations of several people engaged in the work for the blind. In 1929 U.S. Senator Thomas D. Schall, who was blind himself, proposed a bill in Congress allowing blind people to operate vending stands in public buildings. But the bill was defeated, as was a similar one in 1933.

Despite these reverses, the advocates of the vending stand legislation continued their campaign. Aided by the relentless and untiring efforts of Leonard A. Robinson, a blind attorney from Cleveland, Ohio, the stand lobby sought additional Congressional support. In 1934 Robinson met Congressman

Jennings Randolph of West Virginia at a Lions Club convention and as a result of this encounter Congressman Randolph became a powerful sponsor of the proposed program. A former Lions District Governor, Randolph had been active in the club's sight conservation program for several years. At the beginning of 1936 he introduced a vending stand bill in the House, while Senator Morris Sheppard proposed a similar piece of legislation in the Senate.

A year after the Randolph-Sheppard Act became law, a fascinating individual named Joseph Clunk became the project's first administrator, and as Frances Koestler wrote in her excellent study, *The Unseen Minority*, Clunk became the "right man in the right place at the right time." Blinded as a young adult, Joe Clunk's indefatigable spirit had enabled him to overcome many of the limitations of his handicap. After selling toiletries door-to-door, he had been a staff member of the Cleveland Society for the Blind in Toronto, Canada. He spent the next nine years establishing a vending stand and industrial placement program for the blind of Canada before becoming the administrator of the stand program in the United States. Over the years I worked closely with Joe and we became good friends. I don't believe I ever met a more zealous and talented advocate of the blind than Joe Clunk, and I believe that much of the success of the vending stand program is directly attributable to his outstanding leadership.

Under the previsions of the Randolph-Sheppard Act, each state established a public agency to license the new vending stand operators and supervise their training and placement. The licensing agency also had the responsibility of finding local sponsors, recruiting blind operators and locating public buildings in which a stand could operate.

In Arkansas we wanted the legislature to create a separate commission for the blind, but when the proposed legislation failed we tried to influence an established state agency to assume the responsibility of coordinating the new program. After the head of the Vocational Rehabilitation Department rejected the project, the chief of the Welfare Department reluctantly agreed to allow his office to act as the licensing agency and by the spring of 1939 the state was ready to inaugurate its first vending stand program. I was flattered when Welfare Commissioner John R. Thompson invited me to his office and offered me the position of supervisor of the new program.

Ironically, I was not particularly interested in the job at the time. I had my law degree, my license to practice law and had every intention of pursuing a legal career with perhaps a venture or two into the political arena. But at the same time I was impressed with the possibilities of the vending stand program. In fact, the previous spring I had delivered a speech to the annual meeting of the Arkansas Association for the Blind (I served as the president of the group that year) urging that the Welfare Department assume the duties that would normally be conducted by a commission in securing employment for the blind.

I believed strongly in the employment opportunities for the blind who could not have their sight restored and the *Arkansas Gazette* agreed with me in an editorial on my address. The editorial writer said that "a state commission, as Roy Kumpe proposed, could meet a real need and render services of the most practical as well as appealing kind." Mr. Thompson had heard my remarks and consequently offered me the new position. Because I believed I could have a genuine impact in a relatively brief time, I accepted his proposal and launched my professional career in the work for the blind. Intending to stay six months at the most, I never dreamed the work would expand so rapidly or become a lifelong obsession.

That June I assumed my responsibilities as the supervisor of the state's new rehabilitation program for the blind. Immediately I began contacting civic organizations to act as sponsors, recruiting blind vendors and working with local officials to establish sites for the stands. I vividly recall the speech I delivered again and again that summer; upon reflection, I realize the theme of that address has remained the cornerstone of my career. "The blind do not want the pity or the sentimental gushing of sympathetic people. They want to work and be self-supporting. Eighty-five percent of the blind in Arkansas lost their sight after they turned twenty-one and these are restless and uncomfortable individuals who wish with all their hearts they had steady employment so they might benefit rather than hinder the world."

I worked closely with Joseph Clunk throughout the summer and with his advice and aid, by August I had created the Arkansas Employment Service for the Blind, Inc. The AESB functioned as a non-profit corporation, with the Welfare Department funding the administration of the program and Vocational Rehabilitation paying a fee to offset the cost of training blind people to operate the stands. The AESB sought loans to establish the stands and the corporation, not the operators, repaid the loans. The Welfare Department, as the licensing agency, had to secure a location, select a blind person to be the operator and furnish the equipment and original stock.

We also adopted a constitution that provided for a set number of board members, including the three state officials who were directly involved in the services for the blind: the commissioner of welfare, the superintendent of the state school for the blind, and the director of vocational rehabilitation. I wanted to include these people on the board to insure that the program would always maintain close ties to the other agencies involved in rehabilitation. Even then I recognize the need for cooperation among organizations involved in helping the blind. We all had the same goal — to help every blind person fulfill his or her own potential — and so I hoped to minimize conflict by including these individuals in the decision-making process in the new program.

Under this system our first vending stand opened at the state Welfare Office at Little Rock on August 26, 1939. We selected Earley Busby, a young graduate of the Arkansas School for the Blind, to operate the stand. For several years he had tried to support his blind wife and infant daughter, but until the stand opened his only income had been from the sporadic sale of brooms and a small "aid to the blind" check from the Welfare Department. To him, the stand represented an opportunity to demonstrate his own competence and become an independent, self-sufficient member of society.

This stand at the Welfare Office became a showcase for the program and soon after it opened I began traveling the state to recruit blind operators and establish new stands. Filled with enthusiasm for the new project, I could never have anticipated the obstacles I encountered that year. Whenever I located a visually handicapped person who seemed eager to become a stand operator, the family usually opposed the idea. They didn't believe their blind relative had the ability to manage a vending stand on his own. The blind person had always been so helpless, passing the days in a rocking chair on the front porch or hidden away in the back bedroom. Many blind individuals had lived this way for ten or fifteen years.

I remember one particular case near Monticello in Drew County. I had a difficult time locating a prospect until I heard about a blind man who lived out in the country. He shared a tiny farmhouse with his wife and parents and when I arrived I found him sitting alone on the front steps, spending the day in idleness as he had done every day since he was blinded ten years earlier. I talked with him for a while and discovered the only thing he had done during that decade that he considered productive was the one day his family had allowed him to "pick off" peanuts. He had been able to pick off as many as some of the sighted members of the family and he talked endlessly about the event as if a miracle had occurred.

After I explained the stand program to him, he seemed willing to try even though the job necessitated moving into Monticello. I helped him find a new home in town and the first day the stand opened his wife dutifully brought him to the courthouse. She found a chair in a far corner of the building for him and then went behind the counter to wait on customers. When I told her that was her husband's job, she pursed her lips into a tight line of disbelief. "He can't work," she said, "He's blind. Blind people can't work." I had a difficult time convincing her I could teach her husband to operate the stand by himself. Even after I got her to agree to go home, she only went across the street to see what would happen.

After ten years of being told he was helpless, the man had no confidence in his own abilities. Gradually I taught him how to identify money, how to keep his stand clean, how to order and display his stock. I instructed him to rotate his goods to avoid selling stale or spoiled items. Most importantly, I tried to impress on him the idea that his stand had to be tidy and well-operated. I did not want people to buy from him because he was a poor blind man. I wanted them to frequent the stand because it offered quality merchandise in a well-run place of business.

Slowly my efforts began to pay dividends. The man learned to operate the stand and, as an employee of the AESB, he became self-supporting and functioned as a productive citizen of his community until the end of his life.

Overcoming the family's initial skepticism was only one problem in recruiting stand operators. Another barrier was the fact that many blind people feared they would lose their monthly check from the Welfare Department if they took a job. Although only a small check, the money represented a contribution to the family's well being and they had a horror of losing it.

In rural areas blind people were often "hidden away" — the result of some popular myths surrounding the loss of sight. One predominant notion I encountered was that blindness is a punishment for some past sin. Parents of blind children often confessed to me they believed their child's condition was God's retribution for their own misdeeds. Again and again I heard otherwise intelligent people, in referring to a blind citizen of their community say, "I can't imagine what he did to deserve that."

Many people also had the opinion that unless a person lost his sight in an accident of some kind, he probably went blind as a result of venereal disease. In those days guilt and shame played an important role in ideas about blindness. Loss of sight meant evil and darkness. Those being punished were forced to grope in the dark.

Unhappily, these images of blindness are not limited to rural areas but too often persist in more sophisticated segments of society, perpetuated by the mythology, literature and Biblical stories of western civilization. For example, the ancient Greeks often murdered blind infants, assuming they would always be a liability to society. This bizarre practice received the approval of both Plato and Aristotle, two of the western world's most eminent philosophers. In Sophocles' famous play *Oedipus the King*, at one point the chorus summarized many individuals' attitudes on blindness by saying "thou wert better dead than living and blind." Even the Bible contributes to these uninformed attitudes characterizing blind people as groping, stumbling and unable to find their way. (Deuteronomy 28:28-29).

In my travels I found many sighted people who regarded all blindness as a contagious disease and constantly avoided recently blinded friends or relatives. Most people scoffed at the idea that the blind individuals in their community could ever be anything but objects of charity and some even told me they thought it would be cruel to make blind people work.

Thoughout the winter of 1939-1940 I crisscrossed the state of Arkansas combating these myths and opening new stands. I spoke to hundreds of Lions Clubs, Kiwanis Clubs, Rotary Clubs and other civic organizations. I visited every county in the state, soliciting the aid of county and municipal officials who would allow us to operate a stand in the local courthouse. Joseph Clunk told me the program in Arkansas would be regarded as a success if I could have six or seven stands in operation within a year. By the fall of 1940 there were sixteen stands in the state, all showing a profit. I was hooked. I believed in the program. I believed that blind people could learn to be self-supporting and independent. I also regarded the stand program as only a beginning. I could see unlimited possibilities for other programs and I wanted to be a part of any future expansion in the rehabilitation of the blind.

Some of my enthusiasm for my "temporary" career also stemmed from personal encounter with the incomparable Helen Keller. In October, 1939 state officials scheduled Miss Keller to appear at the dedication of the new state School for the Blind on Markham Street. As president of the school's alumni association, I served on the dedication committee and joined superintendent Finis Davis in greeting her on arrival at the old Union railroad station. We met Miss Keller on the platform and when I was introduced she said, "Oh, Mr. Kumpe." She spoke in a monotone and pronounced my name "Koompah." Then she said, "We know about you and we are glad that you are starting a program for the adult blind." I could not have been more flattered — a young man who had only been working in the field a few months receiving recognition from one of the most inspirational figures of the twentieth century.

We escorted Miss Keller and her secretary and interpreter, Polly Thompson, to their suite at the Albert Pike Hotel. Miss Thomson had assumed this position when the famous Anne Sullivan Macy had died a few years earlier. A delightful person in her own right, Polly Thomson kept Miss Keller informed of the conversation by forming symbols and letters in her employer's hand. The entire afternoon melted into an enjoyable and stimulating experience and I marveled at Miss Keller, imprisoned without sight or hearing, enjoying a cocktail, laughing at a joke or commenting on various remarks by others in the group.

We all felt Helen Keller's presence gave the school's dedication a highly special significance. During the ceremony Governor Carl Bailey delivered a rousing speech but just as he reached the point where he was to introduce Miss Keller rain began to fall. Although the governor continued to read his notes until the ink ran all over the page, we had to move the proceedings into the school's auditorium. Because the indoor facility had a seating capacity of only around two hundred and fifty people, many of the several thousand persons who had come to hear Miss Keller speak had to miss the opportunity of hearing her.

Since I had already visited with our guest and wanted to give other people a chance, I didn't attempt to get inside the auditorium. Several friends told me she rendered a wonderfully inspirational address despite the fact that the heat and humidity inside the auditorium became suffocating. I vividly remember that when the dedication ended, and people emerging from the building seemed more soaked from perspiration than those who had remained outside in the rain.

That evening I attended a dinner for Miss Keller at the Albert Pike Hotel and again found her to be an exhilarating person. Although a socialist politically, she believed in self-help for the handicapped and she made a comment quite applicable to my own work that night. "The blind do not want charity," she said, "They want useful work and their share of life's sweet accomplishments."

During my student days at the school for the blind we often debated which was the most serious handicap, deafness or blindness. Of course we always agreed that deafness was the worst. But when I saw a person who had both handicaps and yet who graduated from college, who had been able to free a mind that might have otherwise been trapped forever, I drew encouragement for my own pursuits much as a plant draws its strength from the sun.

Actually Helen Keller was not the only woman who influenced my life in 1939. In my last year of law school I visited the office of Municipal Judge Harper Harb because in those days a municipal judge could decide who represented an individual in court and that individual did not always have to be a licensed attorney. I had a potential client who had asked me to represent him and so I went to the judge's chambers to seek his permission. The judge had an attractive secretary named Berenice Gray and I will have to confess that, after meeting her, I was in no particular hurry to talk to Judge Harb.

When I did get in to see the Judge he agreed to let me serve as the attorney for my client in his court. While I was certainly excited about this turn in my career, I found myself dreaming up additional excuses to visit the Judge's office again. Finally as manager of the ArkLaw Yearbook I decided to ask him to sponsor a page in our annual. When I returned to the courthouse the Judge could not see me. (I learned later he was taking his nap) and Miss Gray and I had a nice visit. She told me to leave my material and she would make sure Judge Harb purchased the ad. When I came back a couple of days later, sure enough, she had secured the money.

I found out that Miss Gray liked to dance and several months later, after I received my first fee as an attorney I invited her on a date. We attended a legislative ball at the old Rainbow Garden in the 555 building, where we shared a wonderful evening. Enjoying each other's company, we danced the night away and Berenice and I have been dancing ever since.

We were married over the Thanksgiving holiday in 1939 and left immediately for Jonesboro where I had to open a new vending stand. The town featured a nice hotel and we honeymooned on the state expense account. At that point I realized my life was taking on a sharper focus. I had a partner with whom I could share my dreams and I had found a new career in the field of rehabilitation.

Within a few years, however, the vending stands became more of a challenge than I had anticipated. With the coming of the Second World War, keeping the stands operating became increasingly difficult. Every necessary commodity seemed to be in short supply. In pleading with our jobbers and other people for special quotas, I never made my request on the basis of sympathy. I argued instead that they were going to have less and less to put into the civilian market because the War Department had requisitioned fifty percent of their products to go to the Armed Forces canteens. I reasoned that all of our stands were located in public buildings where the traffic would always be heavy and the stock could be more easily distributed and I knew that a lot of small out-of-the-way filling stations and tiny grocery stores would be forced to close for lack of gasoline or rubber. Most of the suppliers agreed and as a result, the volume of sales from the vending stands actually increased during the war.

In 1943 Congress voted to amend the vocational rehabilitation statutes by enacting a measure sponsored by Representative Graham Barden of North Carolina and Senator Robert M. LaFollette, Jr. of Wisconsin. The resulting Barden-LaFollette Act (Public Law 113) drastically altered the whole concept of vocational rehabilitation to such a degree that the legislation is often referred to as the Magna Carta for agencies for the blind. The original act of 1921 only provided for payment for vocational training. The new act made available funds for physical restoration and prevocational training services that made the physically handicapped person capable of engaging in remunerative employment.

From the standpoint of the blind in Arkansas, the Barden-LaFollette Act had an immeasurable impact. The vending stand program immediately expanded because the act provided for tools, merchandise and other equipment.

Finally, the new legislation created the Office of Vocational Rehabilitation (OVR) under the Federal Security Agency. In Arkansas my office then shifted from the Welfare Department to Vocational Rehabilitation in the Department of Education. My main function remained the supervision of the stand program through the Arkansas Employment Service for the Blind, but after 1943 I expanded the program into private buildings as well as public ones. We had already demonstrated that blind people were productive workers and therefore hoped to establish new locations in office buildings or industrial plants that wanted food service.

One problem we were able to solve during this era was the inability of blind people to qualify for health insurance. Up to that time, insurance companies apparently assumed that blind people had more accidents than their sighted counterparts and were therefore poor insurance risks. By presenting factual data, including the safety records of blind workers, I convinced Lincoln National Life Insurance Company of Ft. Wayne, Indiana to accept a proposal for a group life and hospitalization policy for the stand operators. This proved to be a pioneering effort in that other blind groups were soon to purchase similar policies.

Besides creating the stand program in Arkansas, I successfully promoted a bill in the state legislature in 1944 to fund home teaching for the blind. Now called rehabilitation teachers, these home teachers were blind persons who visited the homes of newly blinded individuals and offered counseling and some basic life adjustment instruction. Finally, I also began locating jobs for blind people in defense plants during World War II. Many of these positions were highly skilled and paid excellent wages. Gradually I realized I had more opportunities than I had competent blind people. This situation became increasingly frustrating because I knew that numerous blind people could have handled those jobs if they had some kind of prevocational training. They needed to learn mobility in order to travel independently back and forth from work and many needed to improve their communications skills. I recognized the extent of this problem when I tried to recruit several blind people to come to Little Rock to train for the stand program. I discovered that the people who ran the local hotels and boardinghouses did not want blind lodgers. They were afraid blind people might start a fire or need someone to take them to the bathroom.

Out of this experience an idea occurred to me — what if we set up our own boardinghouse? What if we staffed it with people who understood about blindness and could teach the blind people who came there about how to get along in the city? The idea seized my imagination like nothing I had experienced before. Unable to sleep at night, I lay awake planning what the new facilities would be like. As I pursued my daily task I realized more each day that blind persons needed to be trained psychologically and socially before they were trained vocationally. From that realization came the dream and then the reality that would shape the next forty years of my life.

CHAPTER 3
Knights of the Blind

My good friend, the late Father Thomas Carroll, once eloquently defined rehabilitation for the blind as the process "whereby adults in varying states of helplessness, emotional disturbance and dependency come to gain new understanding of themselves and their handicap, the new skills necessary for their new state of a new control of their emotions and their environment." This was precisely the concept I envisioned as I began trying to make my idea of a rehabilitation center in Arkansas a reality.

Drawing on my experience in the field of rehabilitation, I felt the center should be an extension of the vending stand program organized as a non-profit organization rather than as a state agency. Because of my success with the Arkansas Employment Service for the Blind in establishing the stand program I believed the same principle could easily be applied to the new project. A private enterprise could operate with the efficiency of a well-run business while avoiding the excessive regulations and bureaucratic entanglements that seem to ensnare so many state agencies. I also liked the private corporation concept because I knew there would not be enough blind people in Arkansas alone to justify the center and by being a non-profit organization, the institution could supply services to blind clients from neighboring states as well.

My final argument for the private approach involved the availability of training fees through the vocational rehabilitation provisions of the Barden-LaFollette Act. In other words, the rehabilitation center I envisioned would function as a non-profit agency providing services paid for in part by fees from the state. To me, that concept reflected the best of all possible worlds.

I already knew what a rehabilitation center could accomplish through the work of the U.S. Army's Old Farms Convalescent Hospital in Avon, Connecticut. Modeled on the post-World War I English facility, St. Dunstan's, Old Farms helped train American soldiers blinded in the Second World War. The term "hospital" was a misnomer since the services offered at Old Farms were closer to those of a training school for the blind. While I realized we could never duplicate the services of a federally sponsored program in Little Rock, I believed Old Farms did provide an important pioneering effort in organizing an adjustment center for the blind.

Consequently, during the summer of 1946, I visited Avon to tour the facility I hoped would serve as a model for my proposed center in Arkansas. Housed in a boys' prep school in the beautiful Farmington River Valley, Old Farms reminded me of a gigantic English manor house with its rock walls and exposed ceiling beams. Under the command of Colonel Frederick Thorne, an ophthalmologist for the Army Medical Corps, the Avon center stressed self-care and personal adjustment, physical exercise, social recreation and various improvement courses like Braille, typing and music. Through a lengthy testing process the Old Farms staff also tried to identify vocational aptitudes and interests on the part of their blind patients.

I spent two days at Avon under the tutelage of a counselor I had met earlier through the American Association of Workers for the Blind. One of the first things I noticed as we toured Old Farms was the strong emphasis the staff placed on mobility. For the first time in my life I observed the work of an individual trained to teach a blind person the use of a cane as a mobility aid. My friend called these people "orienters" and showed me how they took the blind soldiers around the campus grounds and taught them to use the cane in a rhythmic sweeping motion. The agility of many of these soldiers went far beyond anything I had witnessed in Arkansas.

The staff also included braille instructors, many of whom were blind themselves, and specialists who taught typing and other communications skills. My initial impression was that the employees outnumbered the trainees, which later proved to be true; the Avon facility had a better than one-to-one staff-patient ratio. From my first moment at Avon I recognized that we would never be able to duplicate in Arkansas the homogeneity of the trainees at Old Farms. All of these young men had served in the Army; all had been blinded suddenly by an accident; and all of them were young enough to have the faith their lives could still be productive despite their handicap.

Since the war had only recently ended, numerous trainees were blinded prisoners of war from Japan. Several of these men had participated in the grisly Bataan "Death March" and most of their blindness had resulted from malnutrition rather than shell explosions or other violent war wounds. For the first time I realized that the lack of a proper diet could cause blindness. Years later when I began helping the governments of developing nations inaugurate progams for their own blind I drew upon this earlier experience and pointed out that many people in these emerging nations had been blinded by malnutrition and a new emphasis on diet might reduce the number of sightless individuals.

A final thing that impressed me about Old Farms was that, as an army facility, all of its procedures rigidly followed military discipline. The staff forced all of the trainees to pass through a mess line at each meal exactly as they would have done in the regular army. I thought it most inconsiderate to force these men to suffer the humiliation of trying to carry a tray full of food while they felt their way to a table. When I asked the director why the institution maintained that ridiculous policy, he shrugged and said, "Well, we're part of the Army and you just can't get those regulations relaxed." Although I learned numerous valuable lessons about running a rehabilitation center from my trip to Avon, military compassion and military logic were not items I wanted to transplant to the new center in Arkansas.

After my tour of the Avon facility I made a brief excursion to New York City to visit an old friend in Manhattan. In the immediate postwar era hotel rooms were difficult to find in New York and the only accommodations I could locate cost twenty dollars, which was far more than I could afford. My friend told me not to worry about the room. He telephoned the headquarters of the American Foundation for the Blind and the kind people there found me a comfortable room for only five dollars a night. When I called Dr. Robert Erwin, the director of the Foundation, to thank him, he graciously invited me to lunch. One of the early giants in the work for the blind, Robert Irwin had been active in the formation of the AFB and had served as its director for many years. People in the field of rehabilitation usually mentioned Irwin's name with awe.

We lunched at an exclusive private club near Park Avenue and toward the end of the meal I began to tell Irwin about my trip to Avon and my plans for a rehabilitation center in Arkansas. Instead of the enthusiastic approval I expected, Irwin shocked me. "Ah, there's nothing to that," he signed. "You're just starting another home for the blind. It's all been tried before. It won't work."

I would probably have felt more comfortable if he had thrown a glass of water in my face. "Well, Dr. Irwin," I responded. "The project could never become a home because part of the financing would come from the Barden-LaFollette Act. Vocational rehabilitation would pay for prevocational training so we could only bring people into the residence who were on a rehabilitation plan and they would have to move out to a job before we could bring in someone else."

Irwin insisted the idea would never succeed because a similar plan had· been tried during the First World War and had failed. I saw little point in pursuing the argument and even though I greatly admired Robert Irwin, I refused to be disheartened by his remarks and I left New York still confident that in the near future I would find the way to build the first rehabilitation center for the civilian blind in Arkansas.

When I returned to Little Rock, I began to organize the initial financing of the project. Because I wanted to expand the voluntary agency I never considered asking for funding from the state legislature. Instead, I launched what I regarded as the key ingredient in my plan — I suggested my local Lions club become a participant in establishing a regional adjustment center for the adult blind.

I chose the Lions Club because of its long history of aiding the blind in various capacites. Founded in 1917, Lions International was the creation of a Chicago insurance executive named Melvin Jones. Before World War I, Jones had observed that both the Rotary Club and Kiwanis Club had grown from simple luncheon groups to genuine forces in the business world and he wanted to add the concept of service to the business promotion aspect of the earlier clubs. Prior to the war, numerous independent luncheon clubs like the Businessmen's Circle existed, and Jones organized a convention of these associations in Dallas in the fall of 1917. Lions International resulted from that meeting. The delegates derived the word "Lions" from Liberty, Intelligence, Our Nation's Safety and they selected the motto "We Serve" to emphasize the role of community service.

In each community the members of the club joined by occupational classification. For example, a local club would include only one automobile dealer, one insurance man, or one tire store owner. Sometimes that policy produced some unusual results. I remember one instance in Little Rock where the club already included a Presbyterian minister when the superintendent of the Methodist Church, who had been an active Lion in another town moved to Little Rock. Since the club already had a Protestant preacher, some people felt there would be a conflict over admitting the superintendent. They finally solved the dilemma by designating one man as being in the wholesale ministry and one in the retail ministry.

Starting in the late 1940s the Lions Club grew rapidly and the classification system became less important. If a member felt any man would be a good addition to the club, he could sponsor that individual for membership regardless of occupation. Once admitted, a new Lion had to attend the regular meetings. Most clubs' constitution contained a provision that if a member missed three consecutive meetings without a good excuse he could be dropped from the membership rolls. The constitutions usually provided for substituting attendance at another Lions Club meeting, which aided businessmen who traveled a good deal.

Almost from the beginning, the Lions Clubs' major area of service centered on aiding the blind. For many years I assumed this concern probably resulted from the fact that Melvin Jones had a blind sister or brother or someone else close to him and because of that he had steered the club into a strong role in the sight conservation movement. In 1943 I discovered the real reason for the clubs' commitment to the blind. While attending a rehabilitation conference in Chicago that year I visited the Lions International Headquarters. After being announced as a visitor, to my amazement Melvin Jones himself breezed out of his office and volunteered to conduct a personal tour. As we walked through the facility I asked Mr. Jones why Lions were so involved in the work for the blind.

The Secretary General explained that the organization's commitment in that area dated back to a Lions convention in Cedar Creek, Ohio in 1925. At that meeting, Helen Keller had electrified the group by demonstrating her ability to communicate and explaining how she overcame her double handicap of blindness and deafness. At that time Miss Keller was involved in a campaign to raise an endowment fund for the recently formed American Foundation for the Blind, so in her speech she challenged the Lions to become "knights of the blind." After her address several motions from the floor demanded that the club adopt the work for the blind as a major function. The convention went on record as accepting Miss Keller's challenge and making sight conservation and aid to the blind the Lions Clubs' major service activity.

After the Cedar Creek meeting local Lions Clubs sponsored a variety of activities as "knights of the blind": raising money for brailling; recording books and educational materials; purhasing typewriters, radios and canes; underwriting cost of dog guides; buying glasses for needy children; and establishing eye clinics. With this background, the Lions Club seemed to be the logical organization to help establish an adjustment center for the blind. Consequently, I approached my local club about the project in August 1945.

I had belonged to the Little Rock Lions Club since 1940 when I joined under the sponsorship of Hugo Norvell of the Schaer-Norvell Tire Company. I felt honored to be invited to join the Little Rock club, which is the oldest Lions Club in time of service in Lions International. That spring I traveled to Fort Smith to attend my first state Lions convention and thereafter became an enthusiastic supporter of the club and its activities. Over the next forty years I attended 18 International Lions conventions in places ranging from Nice, France to Tokyo, Japan along with numerous state and district conferences. I almost always wear my Lions pin, and even today I still feel a tingle of excitement when I think that there are over 33,000 Lions Clubs in 151 nations with over 1.3 million members.

My personal interest in the Lions Club actually began during my student days at the School for the Blind when the club donated a braille edition of the *Reader's Digest* to our school library. At that time our library was little more than a depository of surplus textbooks and I remember being excited to have access to some extracurricular reading material. Even today I recall an article about truck farming in Alaska that appeared in that edition of the *Digest*. Being raised on a similar farm, I found the article fascinating and sincerely appreciated the Lions Club gift. In fact, the school authorities designated me to attend a club meeting to formally express the gratitude of all my students. The club met at the YMCA building at Sixth and Broadway and I remember being impressed by those business and professional men who not only helped those in need but also seemed to have so much fun. They introduced me to the "tail twister" and other Lions jokes and I left that meeting with high hopes that someday I might become a part of the Lions fellowship and commitment to service.

For many years after I became a member of the Little Rock Lions Club I enjoyed the comradeship of the Wednesday noon luncheons and the Monday lunch meetings of the major activities committee. Both luncheons met in the old Marion Hotel and provided a unique combination of fellowship and service. Despite a sometimes excessive amount of boosterism in the Lions Club, the organization's dedication to helping the blind made my forty-year membership in the group a meaningful experience.

Soon after I joined the club in 1940, our membership decided to sponsor a vending stand and agreed to loan the AESB $150. This process had been an earlier idea of mine and had become an integral element in financing the stand program — seeking an interest-free loan rather than an outright gift from the Lions and other service clubs and having the clubs execute the interest free note.

My initial opportunity to involve the Lions in the center came in the summer of 1945 when our club's new president, Stanley Combs, appointed me chairman of the Sight Conservation Committee. In that capacity I called a committee meeting in my office in August to discuss various projects that would challenge our organization to become more involved in the work for the blind. My committee included Finis Davis, the superintendent of the state School for the Blind; Dewey Thompson of the Arkansas Optical Company; Howard Cruse, a

42

local banker; R. A. Cook, an automobile dealer and former county judge; and Hugo Norvell.

Prior to this meeting the Sight Conservation Committee had been passive and had limited its activites to the occasional purchase of eyeglasses for the needy school children. I felt that since the Lions Club had accepted Helen Keller's challenge to become "knights of the blind," the time had arrived for our committee to increase its responsibilities. At the August meeting we considered two proposals. Mr. Davis suggested a sight saving class in the public schools where partially sighted children could have access to large print books and receive instruction from specially trained teachers.

I personally presented the second idea, although at the time I did not expect an enthusiastic response from my fellow committee members. I proposed the Little Rock Lions Club promote a statewide Lions Club effort to establish a readjustment center for the adult blind. I recognized my idea represented an ambitious undertaking, especially since absolutely no precedent existed anywhere in the country for such a project.

Much to my surprise, the idea caught Judge Cook's imagination. After my presentation he addressed the meeting. "I like this idea a lot," he said. "In fact, I like it so much that if the Lions Club adopts the project I will personally pledge $250 a year for the remainder of my life."

Judge Cook's enthusiasm impressed Stanley Combs. A new Lions Club president always wants to initiate an innovative project and the ambitiousness of the proposed center appealed to Mr. Combs as well as Judge Cook. We debated the merits of the project through the afternoon and finally, to my delight, the members of the Sight Conservation Committee voted to recommend the establishment of the center as the club's major service activity.

Of course, that recommendation had to be approved by both the Major Activities Committee and the Board of Directors before being offered to the membership. As chairman of the sight Conservation Committee, I personally presented the proposal to the activities committee the following month. Because the center required considerable committement in terms of money and volunteer hours, I faced an inordinate amount of discussion, debate and opposition. At

43

each committee meeting I encountered the same basic objections. Someone always argued the project could not be done because it had never been done before. In the past each local Lions Club had organized its own individual community projects and no one had ever tried to create something that would be coordinated on a statewide basis. Some of our members felt the center should be limited to the Little Rock area under the sponsorship of the local club while others wanted to continue buying eyeglasses and white canes. I spent many hours patiently explaining how the center would have to be statewide because no single community had a sufficient blind population to justify the operating costs. I also appealed to our members' competitive instincts. Why not be the first Lions Club to inaugurate a statewide project? Why not show clubs in other states what could be accomplished through the cooperation of local Lions Clubs?

The second major objection centered around the ill feelings between the urban and rural areas of Arkansas. Several men contended that Lions Clubs outside the city would never contribute money to something in Little Rock. Traditionally, the rural areas resented the state's only metropolitan center and this rivalry hovered over everything from high school football to state politics. (Only a handful of men from Little Rock have been elected governor of Arkansas.) I met this challenge by arguing that I had been all over the state for the past six years establishing the vending stand program and in my travels I sensed a lessening of the urban-rural rivalry. I reasoned that all we needed to do was to convince the local clubs that a statewide facility would be the only way their local blind citizens could receive the needed services of a readjustment center.

Of course some members felt the project would be too expensive; that such a comprehensive program would be beyond the scope of the Lions Club project. I explained that while we would have to provide half of the operating budget, the fees paid by Vocational Rehabilitation would cover the other fifty percent. From the beginning the center would be fifty percent self-supporting and the Lions Club would never have to pay all of the center's expenses. I also explained that the proposed center should not be regarded as a luxury. The law entitled every blind person to rehabilitation services and I

44

challenged our members to establish a facility to provide that assistance.

Over a several-week period I sensed the opposition to the project subsiding and a genuine enthusiasm for the center spreading among our local Lions. Late that fall the board of directors of the club agreed to present a resolution to the state Lions convention, and if the convention adopted the resolution, the Little Rock Club would raise the first $10,000 to lease a building, purchase equipment and pay the utilities for the first year of operation.

The following May the state Lions convention met at the Arlington Hotel in Arkansas's famous resort city of Hot Springs. Since Mr. Combs's term as club president was almost over, our new president, Finis Davis, presented our resolution to the convention. Some months earlier, Finis and I, under the direction of our local board, had met with Albert Demeres, an attorney, and prepared the actual formal statement with all of the necessary "whereases" and "therefores." The convention schedule called for our resolution to be presented on the last day of the meeting, so several members of the Little Rock Club, myself included, spent many hours informally discussing the proposed center with delegates from all over the state. We distributed copies of an article from a North Carolina newspaper about a similar program that had recently started in that state. The North Carolina people had acquired an old Navy facility and received legislative authorization to inaugurate what they called a preconditioning center. The convention delegates in Arkansas liked the article and seemed receptive to the idea of establishing a center in our state. I remember spending many hours on the hotel veranda discussing the proposed project with my fellow Lions from throughout Arkansas and I recall my pleasure as I realized many of the delegates shared my excitement.

One problem that concerned me was the election for district governor. In 1946 Arkansas had only two district governors and the competition for one position that year was especially fierce between a preacher from Stuttgart and a utility company sales manager from Hot Springs. Backed by their respective clubs, both candidates campaigned hard, which placed the Little Rock club in a dilemma. Since both candidates had many supporters, we did not want to offend one group or the other and possibly alienate them from supporting our resolution. We finally solved the problem by having the Little Rock delegates cast secret ballots and avoid public support of either candidate. Edward G. Barry, the utility executive, won the election and his victory, although I did not realize it then, was to provide the readjustment center with one of its staunchest supporters for years to come.

On the last day of the 1946 convention, Finis Davis presented the resolution calling for the creation of a prevocational adjustment center for the adult blind. The statement recommended that the delegates adopt the center as a statewide project and then appoint a committee to conduct a study on how to coordinate the work of all the Lions Clubs throughout the state. Apparently the members of the Little Rock Club had done their preliminary work well. The resolution passed with a minimum of discussion.

I witnessed the proceedings of that meeting with a growing sense of pride and purpose. Those business leaders had taken a bold step in adopting the nation's first statewide Lions project and I believe that they had established a foundation for making Arkansas a pioneer in the rehabilitation movement.

Immediately after returning to Little Rock, our local club set out to raise the promised $10,000 for the building, equipment and utilities. After several meetings we decided not to conduct a public fund raising campaign. Rather, we chose to solicit the majority of our needed funds from the Little Rock business community. The main factor in this decision was the presence of what was then referred to as the "rat money."

The "rat money" originiated during the war when the city's chief public health officer asked the Lions Club to sponsor a program to eradicate the problem of rodents in the city. The presence of the rats created a health hazard but the public health department lacked money to exterminate the creatures on a wide scale. Under the auspices of the Lions Club, city officials created a $10,000 revolving fund to hire trained crews to rat-proof restaurants, cafes, warehouses and other property where the rodents posed a problem. The property owners were more than willing to pay for the service because of the wartime difficulty in finding qualified people to perform this kind of work. The program succeeded to the point that when it ended, the revolving fund remained intact.

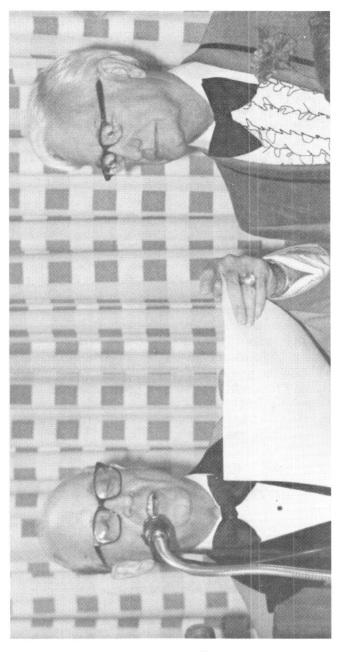

In 1975 Roy Kumpe received the Ambrose M. Shotwell Award from the American Association of Workers for the Blind in Atlanta. Finis Davis, the 44th president of Lions International and vice-president and general manager of the American Printing House for the Blind, presented the award.

47

While the members of the club debated what to do with the money, I tried to devise a plan to use the funds for the adjustment center. Before too long I realized this idea would not work because a growing number of Lions wanted to return everyone's money. They thought this gesture would build tremendous goodwill for the club and to a large extent they were right. We surprised many local businessmen when a delegation of Lions stopped by to refund their contribution. I remember some of them laughing and saying, "Why in the world are you returning this money? I've already written it off my taxes as a contribution."

Less than a year after the refunding of the "rat money" we launched our campaign to raise the $10,000 for the adjustment center. Since we solicited from many of the same people, the goodwill of the earlier campaign really did carry over and these businessmen gladly contributed to our new project.

Under the co-sponsorship of Charles Meyers of Meyers Bakery and George Tyler of First Federal Savings & Loan, the campaign fulfilled all my hopes.

Toward the end of the drive we did make some public appeals and I remember recording a series of brief speeches to be played on the radio. I regarded the whole experience not just as a fund-raising campaign but an opportunity to educate the public to the needs of blind people. The radio broadcasts taught me a lesson in the power of the mass media as an educational tool. For many years thereafter I tried to utilize the radio and television to inform people of our activities at the center and maintain the public interest in our various program.

When we passed the $10,000 mark, I sensed a new era beginning in my own life. The efforts of the Lions Club to promote the new center extended my expectations and I felt confident that under the guidance of the club, the non-profit organizational concept would be able to grow and flourish. I also found exciting the enlarged opportunities for helping newly blinded adults on a regional basis. By the fall of 1946 my dream of a prevocational adjustment center appeared close to a reality. We had the concept, a dedicated organization and the initial funding. The next step was to take this dream and crystalize its physical setting — to locate a place where blind people could come and begin their journey to a new life.

48

CHAPTER 4

To Live Without Sight

What would the new adjustment center for the blind be like? Some people assumed it would be another home for the blind or, since we had teachers, the facility would be another school for the blind. Others believed the center would be a workshop for the visually handicapped or perhaps a small hospital. Actually, from the moment we opened our doors, the Prevocational Adjustment Center for the Adult Blind became a combination of all these elements. The new facility functioned as part home, part school, part workshop and part hospital and most importantly, became an innovative effort to help blind people adjust to their handicap.

Following the Lions Club's successful campaign to raise the initial funds, we set out to locate and furnish a building to house the center. With Mr. Combs serving as our committee chairman we began an exhaustive search for the best available location. I wanted an old residence within walking distance of downtown Little Rock or at least a place conveniently located on the bus line so we could make downtown travel part of our training program.

My bias toward this area stemmed from my student days at the School for the Blind. Back then, the school was situated where the present governor's mansion now stands and I had many fond memories of catching the streetcar or walking to town on pleasant spring afternoons and I wanted the trainees at the new center to enjoy the same opportunities.

Our committee found several excellent prospects in the area near downtown. Unfortunately, no one wanted to rent their property because of the postwar rent controls. We could only acquire a residence in the preferred section by purchasing the property, which the Lions could not afford to do.

After several frustrating months, I located an alternative site in the Oak Forest neighborhood, a newly annexed section in the southwestern part of the city. As a result of a rezoning case on the city council I stumbled on a seventeen-room mansion called the Brack Home on South Tyler Street and Fair Park Boulevard. During the war the house had been used by the United States Bureau of Mines an an office and laboratory for government officials searching for bauxite ore in the area. At the war's conclusion, the place had been abandoned and soon became the victim of neglect and vandalism.

The possibilities offered by this two-story house, which included a floored attic, basement, garage, servant's quarters and substantial acreage, muted my disappointment at not finding a location closer to downtown. I even saw potential in Oak Forest although at that time the sparsely populated neighborhood served primarily as a lover's lane for local teenagers. Oak Forest had grown slowly and the city only annexed the area in the early 1940s. But the neighborhood contained beautiful tree-lined streets and most importantly, the bus company had recently established a line linking Oak Forest with downtown Little Rock.

Mr. W. R. Davis, the operator of a car-wrecking business on the old Hot Springs Highway, owned the Brack Home. During a lengthy series of negotiations, Davis insisted he only wanted to sell the property and not rent to us. Since I presumed his efforts were intended to drive up his rental price, I suggested our committee invite him to join the Lions Club. Davis accepted our invitation and I suspect he thoroughly enjoyed being associated with many of the community's most prominent business leaders. Eventually he agreed to rent us the Brack Home for $250 a month for one year with an option to buy the property for $35,000.

After we signed the lease for our building, the committee began searching for some inexpensive furniture. From a casual remark by a friend from south Arkansas, I discovered that the government wanted to sell all of the furniture and equipment at the Japanese Relocation Center at Rohwer, Arkansas. That facility had been used to house the Nisei Japanese who were so cruelly and unfairly expelled from the west coast during the war.

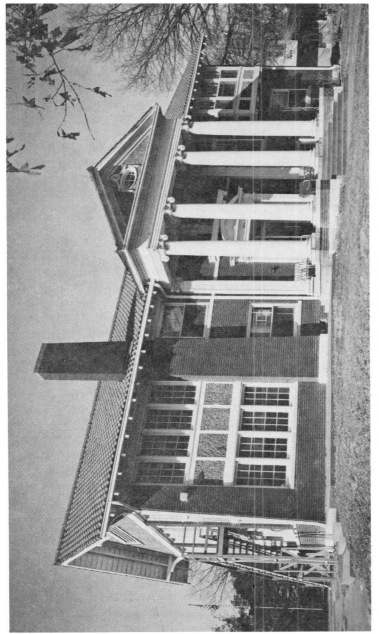

Brack Home, AEB's original home in 1947.

51

I remember Finis Davis, Stanley Combs and I rose before daylight one morning to make the trip to Rohwer to see if any of the equipment might be suitable for our needs. We discovered that a few weeks before the end of the war the government had purchased several maple beds and new matresses for the relocation center but had never used them. That morning we bought fifteen beds and matresses and some other holdings at a ridiculously low price and laughed over our good fortune all the way back to Little Rock.

On January 25, 1947, fifty members of the Little Rock Lions Club swarmed over the grounds of the Brack Home armed with brooms, rakes, shovels and wheelbarrows. They assaulted the debris that cluttered the place, hauled away the trash, replaced the broken windows and prepared the mansion for its new occupants.

That spring the first trainee arrived at the center and on May 5 we held the formal dedication of the Prevocational Adjustment Center for the Adult Blind. If I had to select the most memorable days of my life, that first Sunday in May 1947 would certainly be one of them. The afternoon ceremony took place outdoors in the balmy spring sunshine and the whole day symbolized a great transition in my own life — the beginning of a new era.

Finis Davis, the president of the Little Rock Lions Club, served as master of ceremonies and introduced our distinguished guests, including Arkansas Governor Ben Laney, Little Rock Mayor Sam Wassell and Ashley Ross, the director of the Vocational Rehabilitation Division of the Arkansas Department of Education. Stanley Combs, our club's immediate past president, formally presented the keys to the building to Hugo Norvell, the president of the Arkansas Enterprises for the Blind (the new name of the Arkansas Employment Services for the Blind) and I introduced our guest speaker and my old friend, Joseph Clunk, the chief of the Services for the Blind in the Office of Vocational Rehabilitation in Washington.

In his remarks that day, Joe eloquently interpreted to the public in general and the attending Lions Club members in particular the purpose of our new program. He told all of us that the "loss of sight need not be a disaster to human nature." He also pointed out that we wanted to eliminate the sense of

52

helplessness which inevitably follows the loss of vision. "The public must be made to realize," he said, "that blindness does not result in a lifetime of uselessness and helplessness." I accepted Joseph Clunk's words that day as a personal challenge — to strive to give the trainees who came to our center the tools to begin a new life based on self-confidence and the opportunity to be productive citizens.

Lions District Governor Ed Barry also attend the dedication. During the course of the afternoon, a photographer snapped a picture of Barry, Clunk, the Governor and myself which appeared in the following morning's *Arkansas Gazette*. Ed immediately telephoned me and said, "Roy, get a print of that picture and mail it to the Lions International Magazine." That idea had never occurred to me, but I knew Ed's reputation as a salesman so I followed his advice. As a result, the new adjustment center became the subject of an article (including the photograph) in the Lions Magazine. I appreciated Ed's suggestion, especially since someone from outside of Little Rock had shown such interest in the project.

During those first few months we operated the new facility with an incredibly small staff. In fact, initially we hired only one full-time professional employee — a supervisor. The Welfare Department loaned us a home teacher who worked at the center on a part-time basis teaching crafts, typing and braille and we employed an older couple who lived in the servant's quarters, to maintain the grounds and to serve as the kitchen staff. Of course, I spent as much time as I could spare from my duties with the stand program tending to administrative matters and teaching orientation and mobility at the center.

Even though we stressed crafts such as weaving and leatherwork to teach and evaluate manual dexterity, from the beginning I advocated the installation of a workshop to train people to use both hand and power tools. I thought the shop would help build the trainee's confidence in their ability to be productive in a sighted world. I drew my inspiration for the workshop from Joe Clunk. I had visited the Clunk home in suburban Maryland on several occasions and each time I had marveled at the extensive woodworking shop Joe maintained in the basement. On each trip he showed me some new project

— such as a bookcase or a dollhouse — that he had created with his power tools.

At first my workshop idea encountered some vehement opposition. I remember Stanley Combs, the financial advisor for the center, once told me, "No Roy, I don't want to be a part of buying equipment like that for those blind people. They might cut off their hands or something worse." Stanley's comment typified the attitude of many sighted people. He wanted to help the blind, but he had little confidence in their ability to accomplish much. I persisted in my requests for the money for the shop and tried to patiently explain to Stanley and our other board members how valuable the workshop would be to our trainees.

Finally, Stanley visited my office one day and said, "O.K. Go ahead and buy that stuff. But don't let me know about it, because if one of those blind people has a terrible accident I would always think it was my fault."

I assured him everything would be all right and immediately converted the old bauxite laboratory into a workshop with a lathe and a drill press. Over the years the shop expanded to include a variety of power saws, sanders, drills, bench grinders and other woodworking tools and after thirty years of operation, not one single blind person has ever been seriously injured in the workshop at the center.

At the same time we built the workshop, we also converted the basement of the Brack Home into a home laundry for training purposes and an exercise room where the trainees could pedal a stationary bicycle, skip rope or take a turn on a reducing machine. We believed the ancient Greek dictum of building a sound mind in a sound body applied to our blind trainees as much as it did to their sighted counterparts.

Building those minds and bodies proved to be a difficult task. While I had no illusions of equaling the army's Old Farms program, I did believe that our work could still help blind people who had been deemed non-feasible for vocational rehabilitation. In many ways the center presented an even greater challenge than the Avon project. While the government's job had been to rehabilitate a group of young, reasonably educated and motivated men, civilian centers such as the one in Little Rock received blind men and women of various ages, intelligence levels, educational, social and economic backgrounds and tried to aid them in adjusting to their handicap, often with minimum staff and facilities.

Our first two trainees illustrated the extent of this challenge. Earnest Cheatham, a forty-three-year-old school teacher from Deer, Arkansas in Newton County, had suffered from infantile paralysis, which left both of his legs withered. After attending college he worked as a teacher until glaucoma robbed him of his sight a few years before he came to the center. The vocational rehabilitation people classified Earnest as non-feasible, but he had a positive attitude and we were hopeful our new program could help him adjust to his multiple handicap.

The other trainee, an illiterate man who often joked that he could not remember whether he attended school one or two days in his life, had been blinded in an industrial accident at the Alcoa Aluminum plant. He had done some farm work and WPA-sponsored road work before finding employment in a defense plant. While working for Alcoa he had been unable to read the directions on a lever and consequently had twisted the wrong valve, releasing a torrent of acid directly into his face.

He wanted to open a small grocery store, but I had little hope for his success, especially since his wife was also illiterate. Nevertheless, I personally taught him orientation and mobility and tried to design an individualized program at the center that would meet his needs.

After four months of training, Earnest Cheatham returned to Deer, resumed his teaching post and taught the necessary five years he needed to qualify for his teacher's retirement. He then moved to Walnut Ridge, where he taught for a while at Southern Baptist College. Our illiterate trainee learned the necessary skills to open and operate a home laundry in Malvern, which he used to support his family for twelve years before his death. The success of these two individuals — our first trainees — gave me great hope and inspiration for the future. The concept of the center as a statewide Lions project seemed sound and we had proven that we could rehabilitate at least some "non-feasible" individuals.

During that first year the adjustment center offered training to eighteen people from Arkansas, Louisiana, Missouri, Oklahoma and Tennessee and served as a learning laboratory for all of us. Since we had no models to copy, we had to learn from the day-to-day operation of the center. I recall on one occasion we brought in an Ozark mountain boy who spent most of his time strumming an off-key guitar and singing mournful country songs in a voice that the supervisor assured me could be heard in the next county. "You just can't imagine how corny this gets," she told me repeatedly.

Soon after the first year this supervisor resigned and returned to her teaching career, which created my first personnel problem. After interviewing several people for the position of supervisor, I began to realize how many sighted individuals are actually frightened of blind people. I found myself assuring some prospective employees, "You never know what your emotional reaction to these blind trainees will be, but I want to promise you that you can't catch blindness."

As our new program developed during those early years I added some additional staff members to the center, including a fascinating individual named Jack Kinney. Jack originally came to Little Rock from California to study our center with the intention of starting a similar project in his own state. But in February, 1948, he accepted a position as the training director at the AEB's Prevocational Adjustment Center.

An army pilot during World War I, Jack had later become a successful executive with a Pacific coast oil company. Then, while flying a private aircraft near the California-Oregan border, he had been injured in a plane crash that left him permanently blind. "When the doctors informed me of my loss of sight," he later told me, "the crushing feeling of utter despair is impossible to describe. I felt totally and completely lost. Self-destruction became a constant thought."

Jack resisted his suicidal urges and exiled himself to a remote desert region in Death Valley, California. He had a simple philosophy — he would learn to survive and live as a blind man or he would die. He not only survived his self-imposed ordeal but taught himself to cook, clean and perform other household chores. He emerged from the desert as a well-adjusted handicapped individual.

During the years he worked for the center the staff and trainees called him "Happy Jack" and I have rarely encountered an individual with a more positive outlook on life. In discussing an incoming class he loved to say "This looks like a good group, Roy. We'll send them back with chins up, shoulders back, self-reliant, freed from the fear of being a tax burden." At the center he directed our training program, taught orientation and mobility and helped the trainees learn to do things like eat in public without embarrassment. Along with these duties Jack devoted countless hours to traveling around the state speaking to Lions Clubs and promoting our program by telling the Lions what we were accomplishing and what we planned to do in the future with their help. He educated this audience to the nature of blindness, good-naturedly commenting that to a blind man, "all women are beautiful, all lawns are trimmed and all houses are newly painted." Jack always closed his speeches by saying, "I'll be seeing you again," and I'll always be thankful the center had such a dedicated and inspirational figure to deliver our message during those early years.

We were also fortunate to have Ed Barry aiding our cause in that crucial formative period. As District Governor, Ed traveled south Arkansas and later as the first chairman of the Arkansas Lions Committee for Sight Conservation he toured the entire state speaking to Lions Clubs and telling the story of the center. Everywhere he spoke his enthusiastic spirit seemed to be contagious. Ed loved the Lions Club and in 1950 he decided to run for the board of directors of Lions International. I helped plan his campaign, even though I could not attend the convention in Chicago that year. When Ed won the election he gained a national platform from which he continued to promote the center.

A few years later, Ed's employer, the Arkansas Power and Light Company, transferred him to Little Rock where he affiliated with our Lions Club. Many of our members plus numerous friends from his tenure on the international board began urging him to run for third vice president of Lions International. A devoted believer in the center, Ed served on the AEB board and always said in his speeches that, "the Lions are doing a lot for the blind but the program for the blind is doing more for the Lions." When he asked me if I thought a campaign for third vice president would hurt the center because the clubs in the state would have to raise money which would not be going to the AEB I told him I thought the publicity would actually benefit our work.

The 1954 Lions convention met in New York City and a strong delegation from Arkansas chartered a plane to insure the best possible attendance to support our candidate for third vice president. Berenice acted as a hostess for the campaign headquarters in the hotel and I made several speeches on Ed's behalf to other state delegations.

The Lions sponsored a huge parade down Fifth Avenue the day before the election and I'm sure the delegates from Arkansas were the only people who welcomed the torrential rains that fell on the city that day. We had earlier passed out plastic umbrellas and when the marchers opened them as a shield against the downpour the office workers in the buildings above saw a sea of umbrellas with the message "Ed G. Barry for Third Vice President" lettered across the top.

The full Lions assembly met in Madison Square Garden with all the hoopla of a national political convention. At my suggestion we convinced my old friend and fellow Lion, Congressman Brooks Hays, to place Ed's name in nomination and the University of Arkansas Band played a series of rousing songs for our demonstration.

Ed won a narrow victory in New York and after serving as third vice president and second vice president, he became the president of Lions International in 1957. In that capacity he traveled all over the world speaking to Lions Clubs and serving as a good-will ambassador for the adjustment center for the blind in Little Rock. Everywhere he went, Ed told the story of what we were doing at the center and I don't think we could have had a better spokesman than Lions President Ed Barry.

We were particularly fortunate when, a few years later, Finis Davis was also elected President of Lions International. I had invited Finis to join the Lions Club in 1940 during his tenure as superintendent of the Arkansas School for the Blind. After he left the state to become the superintendent of the prestigious American Printing House for the Blind in Louisville, Kentucky we remained close friends and Finis continued his interest in our work in Little Rock. I was thrilled the day Finis became third vice president the same year Ed became president. Here were two people in the hierarchy of Lions International who had been instrumental in helping me start the rehabilitation center. During their terms in office both men remained enthusiastic supporters of our work and spread the word of what we were doing to Lions Clubs throughout the world.

To solve the problem of maintaining financial support during the first few years of the center's existence, I promoted a seal sale similar to the Easter Seal campaign. We sold our seals in November, using the slogan "Be Thankful You Can See." The campaign took a tremendous amount of the staff's time, even with help from volunteers and by 1954 I decided the net return failed to merit the cost and effort involved.

At that point we shifted to a quota system for each of the 108 Lions Clubs in Arkansas. I presented a budget to the AEB board, projecting what we would receive from the rehabilitation agencies in training fees. We then divided the resulting deficit among the various Lions Clubs on the basis of the number of members in that club, the size of their city and the amount they had been raising through the seal sale. Each club assumed the responsibility of raising their own quota. Some chose to continue the seal sale, others opted for fund-raising events like spaghetti suppers, minstrel shows, light bulb and broom sales. The change to club quotas steadied our financial system although, as the adjustment center expanded, new sources of revenue became a continuous challenge.

During the course of the center's first year of operation I realized that our training would have to be done on an individualized basis rather than in groups or classes. But this approach required extra staff and additional financing. I convinced the rehabilitation people to increase their fees by explaining they were getting a bargain because the Lions Clubs underwrote part of the cost. I also organized a conference of the rehabilitation directors of the six adjoining states to demonstrate our program and show how we could serve their clients as well as those from Arkansas. Eventually this group organized an advisory board which met annually and aided me in offering the blind people of their respective states the best possible services.

After three successful years of the facility's operation, the delegates to the state Lions convention in 1950 passed a resolution recommending the clubs raise $35,000 to purchase the Brack residence and make the mansion the permanent home of the adjustment center. Following the convention I called a meeting of representatives from various clubs to discuss the anticipated fund raising. During the discussion several men voiced skepticism that the clubs could raise that much money. Finally, Ed Williamson, the District Governor from Magnolia, said, "Oh, hell. If the Lions of Arkansas can't raise $35,000, I'll resign and join the Rotary Club." His remark erased the tension in the room and resolved the issue, leaving everyone with a sense of renewed dedication. Through a variety of projects, the clubs raised over $30,000 and then some of our board members signed a personal note to borrow the rest of the money for the purchase of the Brack property.

By the spring of 1950 my dream of an adjustment center for the adult blind had become an established reality. We had proven that our services could rehabilitate blind people and provide them with new opportunities. After purchasing the Brack Home with the support of the Lions we seemed well on our way to making the center a permanent institution. Our catchphrase, "We teach people how to live without sight," summarized our mission and at that point I could not have been happier with the progress of the center. Unfortunately, I failed to note the dark clouds gathering on this bright horizon and during the next two years my dream had to weather its first genuine storm.

The origins of the center's first controversy dated back to before the war years. After the passage of the Randolph-Sheppard Act in 1936, I approached Ashely Ross, the supervisor of the Vocational Rehabilitation Division of the Department of Education, to assume the responsibility of being the licensing agency for the new program. He referred me to the Welfare Department and as a result, that department ultimately became the designating agent, paying my salary and supporting the stand program.

Over the next few years, Ashley Ross worked closely with our agency, paying the Arkansas Employment Service for the Blind a training fee to train blind people to operate the stands. His department then received credit for rehabilitating blind individuals. When the new Vocational Rehabilitation Act passed in 1943, I assumed the Welfare Department would remain the designated state agency. I even approached the Attorney General to secure a ruling to this effect. Unfortunately, Ross interpreted my action as an effort to take control

60

of incoming federal funds away from the vocational rehabilitation department.

Although Ross, Welfare Commissioner John Pipkin, Ralph Jones, the Commissioner of Education, and I resolved this conflict at a lengthy meeting in 1943, the entire affair left a legacy of latent resentment toward the rehabilitation of the blind on the part of some general rehabilitation counselors. They continued to believe that I had tried to deny them federal funds. As a result of that same meeting, I moved my office to the Education Department where I became the supervisor of the services for the blind.

After organizing the center, I resigned and was succeeded in that position by a former rehabilitation counselor who had been away in the military service. Before the war, vocational rehabilitation only worked with crippled people and my replacement had no experience in working with the blind. After he calculated the number of blind people that needed the prevocational services we offered through the center, he informed Ashley Ross that it would take all of the department's money if he referred blind people to the center.

I assured Ross that many blind people would not accept our services for a variety of reasons and his department had no need to become concerned. But many rehabilitation counselors did become alarmed. These people had always resisted the idea of separate rehabilitation counselors for the blind and harbored long-standing resentments against those of us involved in the work for the blind. At that time the cost of rehabilitating a visually handicapped person amounted to almost ten times the cost of performing the same service for an ordinary crippled person, since paraplegics were designated non-feasible.

Another point of friction between myself and the counselors resulted from my advocacy of a separate state agency for the blind. This idea was not a radical proposition since thirty-nine other states already had similar agencies to insure that the blind received their equal share of rehabilitation funds. A survey conducted by the American Foundation for the Blind supported the concept and suggested Arkansas create a separate commission for the blind. Yet in the Byzantine world of state government, many people viewed a commission for the blind as a threat to bureaucratic autonomy and therefore rendered vehement opposition to the suggestion of change.

This antagonism crystallized after the AEB board helped draft a legislative proposal establishing a separate agency. The rehabilitation people regarded the proposed legislation as a personal attach on their work and marshalled their forces to successfully defeat the measure in the Arkansas legislature despite a "do pass" recommendation by a legislative committee.

This legislative fight, combined with earlier animosities, resulted in the near destruction of the adjustment center. The rehabilitation counselors in Arkansas suddenly refused to refer any more blind people to our facility. They spread rumors to the effect that I kept most of the training fees and our clients did not receive the services we promised. The counselors discouraged blind people from coming to Little Rock and participating in the training at the center. They represented the Department of Education, and their disparaging remarks about a new program were taken seriously. The rehabilitation people's campaign also included a speaker's bureau that gave talks before Lions Clubs throughout the state insinuating the program at the center had failed and that the Lions should find another project to aid the blind.

I refused to allow the center to close because of a vicious campaign by a group of narrow-minded bureaucrats. When our referrals from Arkansas stopped, I went on the offensive, visiting our neighboring states, explaining the center's program to rehabilitation workers and agency heads. The out-of-state referrals increased and we managed to keep enough people at the center to justify our staff and keep the place going. But just barely.

The conflict broke my heart; the blind people of Arkansas were missing the prevocational adjustment training they desperately needed because of the vindictive actions of the counselors. After receiving several discouraging calls from members of my own Lions Club, I called on our board of directors to resolve the situation. Board president Ed Barry called a special meeting of the board at the center in early 1952 and invited representatives of the rehabilitation counselors, the supervisor of the services for the blind and Ashley Ross. We reviewed the history of the controversy and I explained that in order to keep the center operating and providing needed services, we had to have the support of the vocational rehabilitation people. Late in the evening the warring factions agreed to a peace treaty. We agreed to drop the idea of a separate agency for the time being and they promised to refer blind Arkansans to the center for prevocational training. At the conclusion of the meeting I experienced a tremendous sense of relief. The first major crisis for the center had passed, and the settlement of that controversy freed me to return to my mission to promoting and developing more employment opportunities for the blind.

CHAPTER 5
Politics and Business

Rather than confining my energies, the founding of the adjustment center acted as a stimulus to increase my involvement in a variety of activities. Along with developing the program at the center, I launched my political career, established a private business and accelerated the pace of my work in various professional and civic organizations. I remember those years as a wonderful and energetic era, even though ironically, I suffered through the worst disappointments in my life during this same period. Fortunately, time has a way of forcing tragedy into a blurry background while holding life's more joyous moments in sharp focus.

As a young man, I harbored an interest in politics from my acquaintance with political figures like Brooks Hays, and one important motivation for me to attend law school had been a desire to become involved in state politics. During my law school years I also drew considerable inspiration from the career of President Franklin Roosevelt. I regarded Roosevelt as a figure of enormous ability who had never let his own physical handicap deter him from pursuing his goals.

I began my own modest political career with a race for the state legislature in 1938. Soon after graduating from law school, I had become active in the Pulaski County Young Democrats Club and the president of that organization, a fine young man from eastern Arkansas named Lee Ward, and several other friends urged me to enter the race. After many years of dreaming of a life in politics, I did not need much persuasion.

In those days the county used a bizarre system of electing representatives. Instead of campaigning for specific positions, the names of all candidates appeared on the ballot in a single list and the seven who received the highest number of votes became Pulaski County's representatives in the Arkansas legislature. My name appeared on the ballot along with thirty-two other hopeful candidates.

A law school professor had once told a group of us that, since attorneys were prohibited from advertising, a race for the legislature provided a young lawyer with a fine opportunity to meet people and let the public know about his practice. After the campaign started I realized how right the professor had been. I probably should have been called the "Happy Candidate" because I thoroughly enjoyed traveling all over the county, shaking hands, passing out campaign cards and discussing local problems and concerns.

By necessity I conducted an inexpensive campaign — I even had to borrow part of the $75 filing fee. Therefore, I tried to make up for my lack of funding with hard work. I shook hands with potential voters until my own hand became swollen and tender; I talked until hoarseness forced me to relax; and I distributed campaign cards with the slogan "Lucky 13 on the Ballot," in an attempt to get voters to remember my name on the lengthy ticket. In rural areas I stressed my farm background and even ran a small ad in a local farm journal urging the voters to "Have One Farm Boy Among the Seven."

All that hard work paid off — almost. Starting with virtually no name recognition, no experience and little financial support, I finished eighth out of thirty-three candidates, one place short of election. Of course, I felt disappointed to have come so close to victory and friends urged I challenge some ballot box shenanigans in North Little Rock, but overall I regarded my maiden adventure into politics as a success. I refused to contest the election, believing I had laid a positive foundation for my next campaign and returned to my work optimistic about my political future.

Five years later I launched my second foray into the political arena. This time I selected municipal government rather than state politics as my goal. At a Lions Club luncheon during the winter of 1943 I sat across the table from Sam Wassell, a member of the Little Rock City Council. Sam informed me that the incumbent alderman in my ward, Edwin Wilson, had decided not to run for re-election and urged me to seek the position. The idea of being associated with city government appealed to me and after discussing the matter with

Berenice and some friends, I decided to try for the post. Since the campaign took place during the war, I did not anticipate a lot of public interest in the council election and assumed I would be able to conduct a fairly inexpensive campaign.

Immediately before the filing deadline, however, Alderman Wilson changed his mind and announced his candidacy for re-election. Suddenly I found myself cast in the role of a newcomer challenging the city hall establishment. While this situation violated my conservative nature, I decided to continue my campaign. A little later I found particular satisfaction in sticking to my decision when a representative of my opponent offered to reimburse me for all of my expenses if I would withdraw from the race. In those days I had a Boy Scout-civics book view of politics and this offer only spurred me on to try my hardest to win the council seat. I enjoyed the support of many loyal friends who knocked on doors, telephoned people and ran transporation pools on election day and after an enthusiastic campaign, I emerged the winner.

Some of the local newspapers hailed my victory as the triumph of a young reformer over the "City Hall Gang" and I will confess I rather enjoyed my new image. At thirty-three I became the youngest member of the council and since I had no obligations to any special group, I eagerly anticipated serving the best interests of all the people of the city.

The first issues that occupied my attention on the council were zoning and city planning. The work of J. N. Heiskell, publisher of the *Arkansas Gazette*, first attracted my attention to these problems. Mr. Heiskell strongly advocated planning the growth of Little Rock for what he anticipated would be a postwar boom. In many of his speeches and editorials he criticized the work of the city council, which often approved spot zoning (allowing single individuals to violate zoning ordinances).

Upon joining the council I discovered a long-standing feud existed between the aldermen and the city Planning Commission. Consequently, one of my first goals became to promote a better understanding between the two bodies. To that end, I successfully sponsored an amendment to enlarge the commission by the addition of three aldermen. I also proposed that the Planning Commission conduct public hearings on zoning applications before they were presented to the council, not only to educate other aldermen about zoning issues but also to alleviate the popular notion that city government consisted of "deals" behind closed doors.

My interest in city planning continued after I left the council in 1948 and began serving an eight-year term on the Little Rock Planning Commission. In the midst of my tenure on the Commission we promoted a new series of regulations for developers and established the concept that a certain percentage of newly annexed lands would be reserved for playgrounds. During this same era the Commission members urged the employment of the city's first professional planner and began to coordinate municipal planning with that of the county. This later activity resulted in metro-planning, which today enables Pulaski County to avoid much of the unsightly urban sprawl that characterizes so many other growth-oriented cities.

Many progressive critics have seen city government as a festering sore of corruption on the body politic. Throughout my years of service on the Little Rock City Council, though, I found that few of my fellow aldermen fit the stereotyped image of a stupid, corrupt official. Most of them were sincere men who tried to serve the people of their ward as best they could.

During my five years of service on the council (1943-1948), several exciting controversies arose. Probably the most bitter conflict of my tenure involved the city's taxicab franchises. I became aware the cabs were a problem after hearing complaints from several acquaintances of mine who had come to Pulaski County to visit servicemen, who were stationed at Camp Robinson outside of North Little Rock. Complaining that the taxi service in the city had become incompetent and inefficient, my friends informed me that the cab drivers often overcharged them.

I investigated the matter and discovered that while the city had two franchise companies, Checker Cab and Yellow Cab, one individual controlled both of them. I viewed this monopoly as totally unfair to the public and resolved that if anyone applied for another franchise permit I would do everything in my power to see that the council approved it. By coincidence, a few months later a former Arkansan named Fredrick R. Andres submitted just such an application. Much to my surprise, the council's transportation committee stalled the application for over a year. Finally, through some intricate political maneuvers, I forced the committee to submit Andres' request to the council. The aldermen approved the new franchise by one vote.

Through my investigation I discovered that while one individual owned both cab companies, he only paid the franchise tax on one and owed the city $5,000 in back privilege taxes. Even though we collected the money under the threat of legal action, our troubles with the taxicabs continued. Mr. Andres started the Dixie Cab Company with five cabs and was ready to begin business until he discovered he could not purchase any meters for his vehicles. At first I assumed this situation resulted from wartime shortages. Then I discovered the owner of the other cab companies had used his influence with the meter people to delay and perhaps even sabotage the new enterprise.

Acting on my recommendation, the council passed an ordinance providing that the city taxicabs charge only by zones. I knew Washington, D. C. used a similar method with great success and following a long and bitter council meeting, the city of Little Rock abandoned the meter system and adopted the zone concept, which has remained in force ever since.

I was proud of my role in the taxicab conflict and regarded the destruction of the cab monopoly as one of the most positive achievements of the city council during my tenure. While there were other important issues in city government at the time — the conversion from trolley cars to buses, the establishment of one-way streets, and disappointing defeat of the plan for a new airport terminal and the inauguration of parking meters — the solutions to the cab controversy always symbolized to me city government at its best.

Another aspect of my council years that I fondly remember involved my efforts on behalf of the black neighborhood that formed the southern boundary of my ward. Unlike some of my colleagues on the council, I always worked to insure that the black community in my district received equal services such as drainage, street repair and garbage collection. Being handicapped and having experienced discrimination firsthand left me more sensitive to the plight of our black citizens than some of my fellow aldermen.

My experience on the Little Rock City Council taught me several valuable lessons both in regard to human nature and the interworkings of city government. For instance, I learned that special interests can have a corrupting influence on otherwise good and decent people and that some political figures have little concern for the well-being of their community. I also learned that, despite some advantages, a ward system is not the best form of municipal government. Each alderman has a tendency to be overprotective of his own small constituency and neglect programs designed to help the city as a whole. Consequently, some years after leaving the council I applauded Little Rock's decision to adopt a city manager form of government.

By 1948 I felt I had accomplished everything I could as a member of the council. Although my name appeared in the newspapers as a possible mayoral candidate and even though I had enjoyed several brief stints as acting mayor, I believed my political future lay in another direction.

Believing I could do more for the cause of aiding the blind as a member of the state Senate, in 1950 I announced my candidacy for a Senate seat early in order to become the front runner in the election. I hoped to capitalize on my reputation as a reform-minded city councilman and the recognition and favorable publicity I had received for my work with the Rehabilitation of the Blind. For a while I enjoyed the unsolicited support of strangers as well as family and friends and the positive treatment my candidacy received in the newspapers.

Then the other candidates announced for the position: state representatives Max Howell and Bob Riley, and well-known businessman Artie Gregory. The resulting summer degenerated into a typical no-issue, non-ideological local race based strictly on image and perceived popularity, and my own campaign suffered from excessive amateurism and naivete. Refusing to call on wealthy and influencial contributors, I only raised around $4,000 to finance my candidacy. I learned quickly that various special interest groups such as utilities and the education lobby spent tremendous sums on state Senate races. Howell's campaign was well financed as was Gregory's.

I finished fourth in a close contest. In the ensuing runoff election between Riley and Howell I supported Riley, but Howell won the race and for a long time did not forgive me for opposing him. In retrospect, I realized what a tough field of campaigners competed in that 1950 state Senate race. Thirty years later Max Howell is still in the Senate and is regarded as one of the most powerful men in state government. Arkansas voters later elected Bob Riley lieutenant governor and Artie Gregory served several terms in the state Senate after his election to a newly created position in 1952.

During the course of the 1950 campaign I promised Berenice that if I lost I would not run for public office again. She never liked the pressure of being in the political arena: the later hours, the fundraising, and the handshaking. I stuck to that promise although years later I saw several opportunities that interested me. Berenice kindly released me from my promise and told me she would stand by me if I ever wanted to hit the campaign trail again, but I realized I probably never would be a good political candidate. For one thing, my visual handicap prevented me from engaging in the subtleties that successful politicos follow regularly. I could not exchange a friendly wave with people across a crowded room because I could not see them. I used to wear thick eyeglasses and people assumed they corrected my vision. Sometimes friends would tell me, "I saw you in town the other day and you looked right at me and didn't even speak. You can't high-hat your friends like that, Roy."

I also abandoned my political career because I held too many strong convictions. My experience in politics taught me that the most successful vote getters, especially at the local level, are masters at avoiding controversial issues and tend to have flexible convictions about substantial matters.

Though no longer a participant, over the years I maintained a keen interest in Arkansas politics, following the careers of colorful individuals like Brooks Hays, Orval Faubus, Winthrop Rockefeller, Dale Bumpers, Wilbur Mills, and David Pryor. For the student of southern politics I found Arkansas to be a fertile ground for study — though occasionally I still wish the name Roy Kumpe might appear on that list of the state's successful political figures.

Although politics always remained an avocation for me, my business career stemmed from the necessity of supporting my family and educating my children while promoting the rehabilitation of the blind. Ironically, I created my food and vending enterprise as a result of my work with the visually handicapped. In searching for ways to raise additional revenue for the Arkansas Enterprises for the Blind, I learned of a franchise operation called the Automatic Canteen Company of America, which placed vending machines in business establishments. Ordinarily, the owner or an employee group received a location fee from the machines, but in states like Virginia the fee went to the commission for the blind.

I wrote to the company officials, hoping to establish a similar service in Arkansas. They politely declined my request, and said they regarded Arkansas' economy as being too agricultural in nature to justify the automatic merchandising business. They also informed me that the state had a per machine tax which made it virtually impossible for the company to make a profit. I discovered that Arkansas did have such a law, but the legislators had it to tax amusement machines and not merchandise dispensers.

Like most Arkansans of that era, I felt confident that more and more industry would locate in our state in the booming postwar period. I also thought that if I could get the per machine tax altered, there would still be a possibility of using vending machines in places where a concession stand might not generate sufficient income to support a blind person. Consequently, I spoke with state Senator Lee Reaves about changing the tax law. Senator Reaves had begun his career as a teacher at the state School for the Blind and had always maintained an interest in our work. Through his efforts, a bill revising the per machine tax passed the Arkansas Legislature in 1947. The bill provided that machines dispensing merchandise would be subject to a single vendor's license, regardless of the number of machines in operation.

Following the passage of the new law, I contacted the Automatic Canteen Company a second time. In a telephone conversation the company representative told me he liked the new tax structure and offered me the distributorship for the state. When I told him I wanted the business for the Arkansas Enterprises for the Blind he refused, explaining that the company's experience with non-profit organizations had been poor and they wanted to restrict their operation to private businesses.

Automatic merchandising had initially experienced a difficult time because of an unsavory association with pinball machines and juke boxes. Many people therefore associated machine merchandising with gambling. Also, in the early days of the business, operators tended to rely on cheap and often inferior merchandise, but the Automatic Canteen Company wanted to break new ground. Led by Nathaniel Leverone, Automatic Canteen's founder, the company upgraded its equipment and stocked name brand merchandise such as Hershey candy products and Wrigley's chewing gum. Leverone maintained high standards and franchised local distributors for a capitalization cost of around $10,000.

While disappointed that the AEB would not be able to participate in the business, I also recognized the canteen service as a possible avenue to gain the financial security I needed to remain in rehabilitation work. So after considerable thought I decided to incorporate a private, family-owned business. Both my father and my father-in-law bought stock in the new company and Berenice served as treasurer and office manager. We started in 1948 in a small way with a single route man to service the vending machines, but every one of us had great hopes for the future of our tiny enterprise.

I founded the canteen business in the aftermath of a great personal tragedy. In the spring of 1946 our sixteen-month old daughter, Jerre, died of accidental poisoning. We had an older son, Chad, and later were blessed with a second son, Peter, but our loss left deep scars for many years. While no one ever forgets such a tragedy, I think the new business did provide a healthy outlet in which Berenice and I both could concentrate our energies.

Our first machines dispensed candy, chewing gum and peanuts. A few years later we added soft drink machines, cigarette machines, and finally even coffee and sandwich machines. Eventuallly the business expanded to the point that we opened our own commissary to make sandwiches, salads and other foods for distribution through our vending outlets. After introducing our first machines in the Schaer-Norvell Tire Company, we began placing machines in other local businesses. Most businessmen allowed us to install the machines as a service to their customers and employees and many of them generously donated the location fee to the Arkansas Enterprises for the Blind.

As I predicted, the industrial area of Little Rock underwent a period of rapid expansion in the early 1950s and our Automatic Canteen Service benefited from this growth. By installing machines in the new plants of companies like Westinghouse and Alcoa, our company grew to include over ninety employees, including a full-time manager who earned more than I did as the director of the AEB, a fleet of thirty-six cars and trucks and our own headquarters building. By the late 1960s the business annually grossed over a million dollars.

During the infant years of the company I always maintained an excellent relationship with our employees. I personally hired almost everyone and knew something about their families and their background. I did not want Arkansas Canteen Service to become an impersonal corporate monster that treated its employees like tiny, interchangeable parts in a complex machine. Despite my earlier efforts, however, in 1960 I received a formal notice from the National Labor Relations Board that the Teamsters' Union had asked for an election to see if our employees wanted to affiliate with their organization. The fact that the Teamsters would even be interested in a small operation like Arkansas Canteen Service shocked me. After considerable research I descovered that our recent expansion into the Ft. Smith area had barely placed our gross receipts under the jurisdiction of the NLRB and subject to union election.

This was the era of Dave Beck, Jimmy Hoffa and U.S. Senate hearings on labor racketerring, and frankly I wanted nothing to do with the Teamsters' Union. I knew something of the history of the labor movement — the early struggles of the miners and industrial workers of the late nineteenth century; the Molly Maguires and the Ludlow massacre — but I strongly believed the Teamsters of the 1960s were another matter altogether. Especially when they wanted to unionize a small family business like ours.

Almost immediately my relationship with our own employees changed. Many of them hesitated to speak to me. Suddenly, workers I had known for years regarded me with suspicion and several new employees hired by our manager while I was busy with the rehabilitation center treated me with something close to hostility.

The Teamsters won the election by two votes and forced me to negotiate a union contract. Throughout these meetings I noticed the union representative referred to the employees as "our boys." Since I had always spoken of them as "men," I commented that "suddenly our men have become your boys"; a statement he did not find amusing. What *I* did not find amusing was the year long contract I had to sign with the union. In order to meet their demands I had to sell the Fort Smith branch, drop any further expansion plans and in some areas actually reduce our business. As a result, I had to lay off several workers and the whole situation slowly degenerated into an Orwellian nightmare.

At the end of the contract, the employees asked for another election and to no one's surprise the union opposed it. After lengthy negotiations through the NLRB, the U.S. District Court forced the Teamsters to call for a vote. As the election approached, I grew fearful we would lose our whole business. Around the same time a local dairy resisted union organization and one night someone dynamited the owner's plant, an event that drove me to a diet of Pepto-Bismol for several days. Finally, our employees requested another election and when the union realized they lacked support, the union leaders withdrew. But the whole experience set the business back several years and perhaps most importantly, strengthened my resolve to sell the company if an opportunity arose.

Of course, other factors entered into the decision to liquidate my holdings. By the mid-1960s both of our sons had almost completed their education, which had always been one of my main goals in founding the business. Also, the Arkansas Enterprises for the Blind had grown to a point that as Executive Director I had to make a choice. There were not enough hours in the day for me to run a private business and continue with my rehabilitation work. Berenice and I had earlier purchased our parents' stock in the company, so in 1967 we sold Arkansas Canteen Service back to the parent company, maintaining our ownership of the headquarters building.

My venture into private business played an important role in my life. Each year Berenice and I traveled to Chicago for a distributors' meeting or to another city for a trade association convention and those excursions became a significant part of our shared experiences. We planned and worked on the

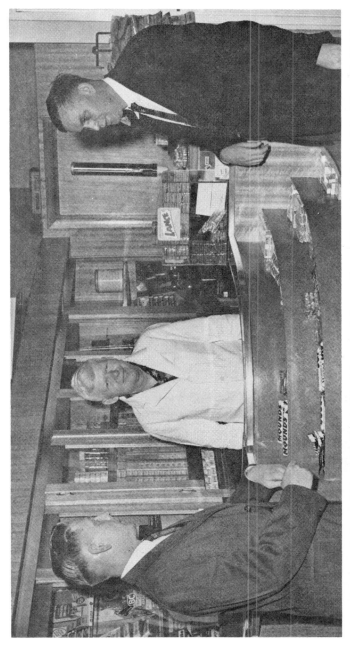

Roy Jackson (left) and E. J. Hall (right) visit one of the early vending stands located in Pine Bluff. They were the first visually handicapped supervisors for the Business Enterprises Program trained by Kumpe. Stand operator is Johnny Boyd.

business together, sharing its successes and setbacks. The company provided the income for my family that the work for the blind could never have done and yet the nature of the vending business left me with the necessary time to serve as the director of the AEB and pursue some of my related interests.

Since the rehabilitation of the blind remained my primary concern, I became increasingly active during the 1940s and 1950s in the American Association of Workers for the Blind. The AAWB grew out of the late nineteenth-century Congress for the Blind, a group founded to promote higher education for the visually handicapped. In 1905 the organization changed its name to the American Association of Workers for the Blind and proceeded to represent all people involved in the profession by sponsoring bi-annual conferences and seminars on different phases of the work for the blind. The leadership of the AAWB defined the organization as an international association which "embraces the layman, the physician, the voluntary worker and the professional worker dedicated to improving the social and economic condition of those who have lost their sight and those with low vision."

My first personal contact with the AAWB came in 1941 when the organization invited me to present a paper on my experiences in establishing the vending stand program in Arkansas. Accompanied by Finis Davis, the superintendent of the state School for the Blind, I attended the AAWB conference in Indianapolis and made the presentation. The AAWB impressed me as a dedicated group of individuals whose goal — to serve the blind — equaled my own. I also liked the group's lack of exclusiveness. The AAWB opened its membership to anyone interested in the cause; not just for special subgroups of those involved in the work for the blind.

Following World War II, the AAWB grew to such an extent that we inaugurated annual meetings. Around that same time the membership elected me to serve on the Board of Directors. After a stint as national membership chairman, I served as the first president and then, in 1951 at the AAWB meeting in Daytona Beach, Florida, the members elected me president of the organization.

In my acceptance speech I challenged our group to actively recruit new, younger and better-educated people to

76

become involved in the work for the blind and to establish our efforts on a. more professional foundation. This challenge stemmed from my overall concern with improving the standards of service offered to the blind people of the nation.

One of my activities as president of the AAWB involved an unsuccessful effort to promote a better understanding between our group and the American Association of Instructors for the Blind. At the time, my good friend, Finis Davis, was the president of the AAIB and he agreed with me that since the interests and goals of the two organizations were so similar they should consider holding joint conferences. But the AAIB board would only agree to a "simultaneous" meeting where the two associations would meet in the same city at the same time but in different locations. Consequently, at our meeting in Louisville in 1952 we exchanged panel programs with the AAIB, but the members of the two groups never met together. This illogical situation was not rectified until 1981 when the AAWB under the presidency of Jerry Dunlap and the Association for the Education of the Visually Handicapped (the new name of the AAIB) under the leadership of Richard Umsted formed an alliance with a joint headquarters in Washington. The goal of the alliance was, of course, the ultimate merger of the two organizations.

Another important issue confronted the AAWB during my term as president — the growing encroachment by federal employee groups on the right to operate vending stands in public buildings which had been guaranteed to blind people by the Randolph-Sheppard Act. This struggle was precipitated by groups like the General Services Administration Employees Organization and the Postal Workers Association installing vending machines in buildings where a blind person might have operated a stand. The employee groups received the location fee and used the money to send flowers to sick members or pay for annual picnics or Christmas parties.

As the AAWB's new president I contacted Brooks Hays, the congressman from my district, who put me in touch with Representative Granham A. Barden of North Carolina, one of the co-sponsors of the Barden-LaFollette Act and the chairman of the House Committee of Labor and Education. After I explained the situation and pointed out how these employee groups were violating the spirit, if not always the letter, of the

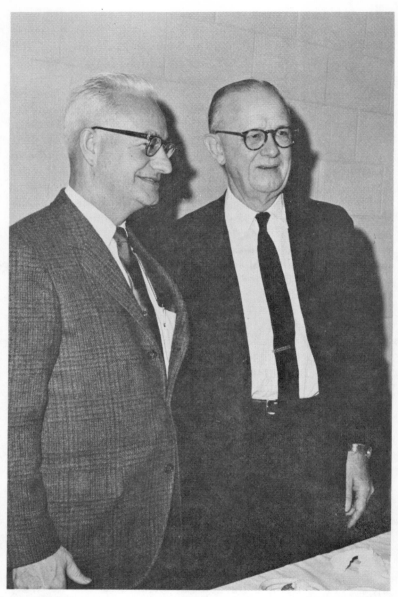

Former Congressman Brooks Hays was a guest speaker at a trainee banquet in 1965. He was a special assistant to President Lyndon B. Johnson at the time.

Randolph-Sheppard Act, Congressman Barden launched a full scale investigation of the matter. Following a series of bitter hearings and meetings at which I suffered considerable verbal abuse from representatives of the employees groups, the situation improved. Although we were unable to secure the legislation we originally desired, the installation of the vending machines in federal buildings sharply declined through an uneasy mutual agreement. The controversy continued far beyond the term of my AAWB presidency and remains a continuous struggle. I know this conflict is difficult for the public to understand because of a general sympathy for the blind and an unwillingness to admit that some people might take advantage of the visually handicapped, but the facts in this particular case seem to speak for themselves.

Along with my AAWB work, my membership on the President's Committee for the Employment of the Handicapped served as an enjoyable outlet for me during the early years of the center's development. This committee grew out of a resolution in Congress in 1948 which designated the first week in October as "Employ the Handicapped Week." At the same time Congress created a presidential committee to promote the special week as well as the employment of the handicapped throughout the year. I received an appointment by President Truman on the committee in 1949 as a representative of the organizations for the blind.

Under the leadership of chairman Ross McIntyre, President Roosevelt's private physician and executive director William McCahill, our committee promoted seminars and conferences, and by the 1980s our annual spring meeting attracted over 1,500 people. A journalist by profession, McCahill had been a Marine in the Pacific theater during World War II and following the war dedicated his life to the service of others. He had a marvelous ability to promote our cause, contacting television and movie screen writers to encourage them to present the handicapped in a positive way whenever possible. McCahill also had our committee sponsor essay contests for high school students and promote the "Handicapped Person of the Year" Award. With his creative guidance the President's Committee became an important force in improving the lives of millions of disabled individuals.

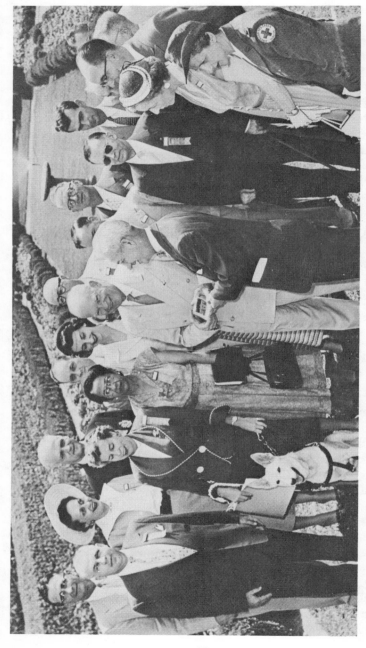

As president of the American Association of Workers for the Blind in 1952 Roy Kumpe met with President Dwight D. Eisenhower in the Rose Garden. Kumpe presented Mr. Eisenhower an AEB ash tray.

Our conferences are always held at the Washington Hilton and have gradually become a trade fair with exhibits sponsored by the manufacturers of aids and appliances for all types of handicapped people. In recent years the committee's main contribution has been the promotion of legislation to remove as many of the physical barriers in public buildings and elsewhere that for years have hindered the mobility of those confined to wheelchairs. I remember Eleanor Roosevelt addressing our group one year and telling us of the difficulties her husband faced when he began his first campaign for governor of New York. She told us of the numerous times he had to be "piped" through a window in order to address a group in a second story hall or auditorium. Through the committee's barrier removal campaign, in the future perhaps campaigning will not be so arduous for other handicapped candidates.

Although overall I am an ardent supporter of removing these barriers, I must confess that, as an advocate for the blind, I am not pleased with some of the recent changes. For example, even though removing a section of curb at each corner makes wheelchair travel considerably easier, a blind person walking with the aid of a cane no longer has an indication he has reached a street corner. I only hope city planners will make some provisions such as moving the ramps off to the side a bit to offset this potential safety hazard.

Years before the President's Committee attacked the problem of barriers, I participated in a memorable occasion involving President Dwight Eisenhower. In 1953 the president entertained a group of AAWB leaders in the Oval Office. After a brief discussion, Eisenhower invited all of us to the Rose Garden for a picture-taking session. In an effort to publicize our new rehabilitation center, I presented the President with a small ashtray containing a picture of our facility. He kept looking at the back of the ashtray while the photographers snapped their pictures, which puzzled me until I saw the photographs. I realized what a considerate thing the President had done by keeping the name and picture of the center in front of the camera.

President Eisenhower strongly supported the President's Committee for the Employment of the Handicapped, endorsing our motto, "It's ability that counts, not disability."

He put all of us at ease at that session in the Rose Garden and at one point said, "Well, I just admire what all of you are doing so much. Keep up the good work."

I felt so relaxed around Eisenhower I instinctively patted the President on the shoulder and replied, "We are so proud of the job you are doing for the country, Mr. President." The next morning the *Washington Post* ran a brief article on the front page that said, "If President Eisenhower had any doubts that he is doing a good job, he has now been reassured by Roy Kumpe of Little Rock, Arkansas."

Those were wonderful and busy years for me. Along with my forays into politics, the canteen business and my work with the AAWB and the President's Committee, I remained actively involved in the Lions Club and taught an adult Sunday School class. But while all of these activities were important, in retrospect, they all seem to have been peripheral concerns. After 1947 the central focus of my life's work became the adjustment center in Little Rock. Even then I realized the center offered the best opportunity to take my dreams and turn them into realities.

CHAPTER 6
New Life

The first years of the adjustment center in Little Rock paralleled the era historians have called the "Great Decade" of expansion of services for the blind. Frances Koestler in *The Unseen Minority* wrote that "few periods in history were as fertile as the 1950s in providing blind people with opportunities and incentives for economic and social progress, [for] ... expanded eductional, vocational and cultural programs availability of jobs and ... new resources for personal adjustment and growth." As early as 1951 I believed our facility had become a leader in that movement.

That same year we changed the adjustment center's name to the Southwest Rehabilitation Center for the Blind. Although the center was still sponsored by the Lions Clubs and operated by the Arkansas Enterprises for the Blind, I felt the new name more accurately reflected the regional nature of the facility. We had also received some criticism that "adjustment" center implied the people who came there were maladjusted. By the mid-1960s we dropped "Southwest" from our name and became the Arkansas Enterprises for the Blind Rehabilitation Center or more commonly, the AEB. No matter what name we used I knew that the important things about the place was not the title on the door but rather the daily activities to aid the blind that went on inside.

During my tenure with the stand program, I identified a few basic skills that I felt were essential for any newly blinded person to possess in order to function in a sighted world. These same skills became the core of our program at the center. While we always emphasized that each blind person is an individual with his own unique needs, we also stressed the mastery of the basic skills for each one of our trainees.

83

The ability to move about independently, a skill referred to as orientation and mobility, has always been a fundamental need for every blind person. When an individual first loses his sight, the loss of the capacity to simply get up and go where he or she wants is a terrifying experience, one that leaves the stricken person with a total feeling of helplessness. I thought one of our own trainees expressed this sensation so well when he said, "You can be a foot away from where you want to be and you're still lost."

For many years I taught orientation and mobility to almost all of our trainees. Using the grounds and walkways of the building, I instructed them in the proper technique of travel with the aid of a cane. Blind people always fear that they are about to step in a hole or stumble and fall. Like sighted people who awaken in the night and try to go through the house without turning on a light, blind people learn to "creep" in order to travel from place to place. Consequently, the basic idea of using a cane is to "clear" a pathway — after you step with your right foot, you use the cane to check where your left foot will be with the next step. The cane also informs the blind person of changes in the texture of the ground, such as a shift from grass to gravel or concrete.

After several weeks our trainees usually develop the confidence to travel with head held erect and not slumped over in the "creeping" position. I also found that this self-reliance in independent travel quickly led to an increased confidence in the trainees' ability to do other tasks as well.

In my lifetime the most dramatic improvement in cane travel resulted from the work of Richard Hoover. A young Physical Education instructor, Hoover served at the Valley Forge Eye Hospital during World War II where part of his assignment included helping orient blind patients to the hallways and teaching them independent travel. Out of this experience, he developed the Hoover Technique of cane travel, which is the basic rhythm method used by almost all blind people today. Not only did he replace the old tapping system, but he also developed a longer and lighter cane which improved travel for the blind. From this experience in orientation, Hoover went to medical school and became an ophthalmologist.

After our first meeting at a conference in the late 1940s, Dr. Richard Hoover and I became friends and I always enjoyed reminding him that the center in Little Rock also made a small contribution to the development of cane travel. One of our trainees, a former blacksmith, developed a system of manufacturing canes from solid Arkansas hickory. He covered the end of the cane with a small spring and hard metal tip which lasted far longer than the old wood or rubber tips. We named the cane the Arkansas Traveler and for many years it was one of the most popular canes in America.

There is considerably more to orientation and mobility than cane travel. For example, we had to teach our trainees to locate items they had dropped on the floor. Many blind people have been injured by bending over and hitting their head on a table or chair. One of the first things we taught in this regard involved protecting oneself by squatting down and carefully exploring the surrounding area for the lost object.

After a trainee gained confidence in his ability to find nearby objects and travel around the grounds of the center, the next phase of training included learning to catch a bus, ride downtown and visit various stores and businesses. During this training we stressed the value of sounds and smells in helping a person travel; locating a bakery, a flower shop, a barber shop, or even a bowling alley by relying on senses other than sight. In 1956 we began the practice of presenting a small winged-cane pin to our trainees who successfully completed their downtown solo. This award has always been a great source of pride and a symbol of growing self-reliance on the part of the blind people who trained at the center.

As part of this solo training we sometimes gave the individual the name and address of another blind person who worked in a downtown stand. Not only did locating these people help our trainees develop confidence, but meeting a blind person, (many of whom were former trainees) successfully working in the downtown area also provided an important morale boost.

As the director of the center, I always enjoyed being on hand when the trainees returned from their downtown solos with stories of their various experiences. Some of the most interesting of these anecdotes involved their encounters with insensitive sighted people. For instance, one fellow related the

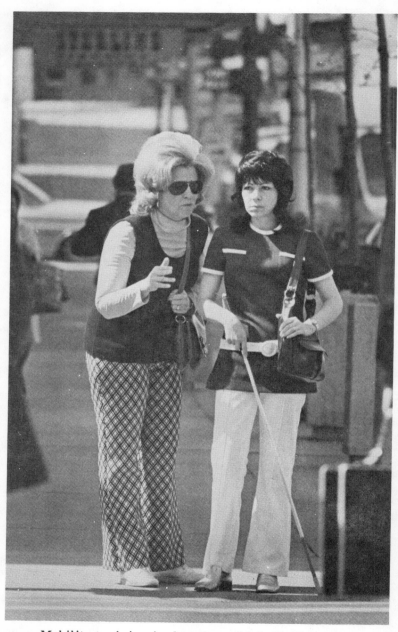

Mobility training in downtown Little Rock — 1974.

story of how he successfully traveled downtown, but while walking around he began daydreaming, lost track of the streets and did not know if he was standing on Louisiana Street or Center Street. He waited until he heard a man approach the corner and then asked, "Pardon me sir, is this Louisiana?"

The man stopped, assumed our trainee was a typical helpless blind man and replied, "Oh no, friend, this is Arkansas."

Another set of basic skills we believed all of our trainees should master involved the fundamental techniques of daily living. For the newly blinded individual, selecting the right tube or jar for grooming needs, going to the bathroom or eating a meal at a formal dinner party are all activities filled with nightmarish possibilities.

To instill confidence in these areas in our new trainees we set aside a forty-five minute period each day devoted exclusively to solving the problems of daily living: how to iron, how to grocery shop, how to mark canned goods for later use, how to use tape to color-coordinate clothing, how to make a bed and care for a dorm room. Blind housewives, of course, needed to learn to cook again in order to regain their self-esteem, so after the first few years of the center's operation we employed a full-time instructor in home economics. The instructor always began by orienting the blind housewife to the stove and other regular kitchen equipment. Years ago the teacher marked the dials on the stove with dots of Elmer's glue using the same principle as a braille watch. After that, our instructors taught the trainees a variety of useful techniques to restore confidence in their ability to cook. For example, the trainees learned to measure liquids with special spoons with the handle bent at a 90-degree angle so the instrument could be dropped straight down into the liquid with a resulting level measure. To prepare an egg for breakfast, our instructors taught the trainees to use a ring cut from a tuna fish can in the center of the skillet as a easily located container for the egg.

One of the most frustrating aspects of being blind is not blindness itself, but rather being forced to adjust to the sighted person's world. Wearing pleasing colors or the latest fashion has little meaning to a blind person, but from the beginning of our training program we stressed the importance to the trainees of making that adjustment. We taught our female trainees to apply make-up by using a blending technique and measuring lotions by a single, quick tilt of the bottle into the palm of the hand. We taught our male trainees to shave every morning using an electric razor and, starting at one side of the face, make a series of concentric circles. The mastery of these personal grooming skills instilled in our trainees an important sense of self-assurance and independence. They learned that they did not have to be helpless and rely on sighted friends and relatives for their basic needs.

A similar situation existed in regard to communications skills. In modern culture the inability to read and write is equated with stupidity and one of our first goals has always been to restore these skills as quickly as possible. One particular young man at the center some years ago had a master's degree, but underwent the embarrassment of being well educated but having to sign his name with an "X". After a few weeks at the center he learned to use a tablet with line guides to enable him to write a legible signature. The restoration of this simple skill changed the young man's entire outlook and encouraged him to work harder at acquiring new capabilities.

The core of our communications program included braille and the use of a typewriter. Our trainees learned not only to read braille but also to write in braille by using a slate and stylus technique. Although a few newly blinded adults ever learn braille well enough to read for recreation, they do learn enough to read and write simple notes or telephone numbers, which reduces their feelings of helplessness.

Finally, for over thirty years the staff at the center has fought a constant battle against the sense of isolation that affects so many of our clients. Many of the trainees had been active people before they became blind but then had withdrawn from family, social or even religious activities. To combat this situation we introduced a recreational program to strengthen their social adjustment skills. We initiated card games such as bridge or pitch or even poker using braille cards. We taught social dancing, bowling and various parlor games. In the days before we could afford a recreational director, our regular staff volunteered to come back on Thursday evenings to lead the social activities. I recall numerous occasions when Berenice and I hosted special recreational evenings in our home. While we enjoyed these pleasant evenings they also served to give our trainees the confidence that they could go into someone's home, participate in a game or other activity, share the refreshments and enjoy the same social benefits as sighted people.

We also found that exercise served a useful function in our overall recreational program. In the old Brack Home, our tiny gym contained stationary bicycles, weights, a punching bag and chinning bars. For years I held the honor of being the champion chinner. I used to challenge the new trainees to develop their muscles to be able to chin themselves as many times as I could. In addition to the other equipment we had a "walking machine" that taught the trainees to abandon the short, choppy steps that so many blind people use and adopt long and purposeful strides.

Like exercise, music often provided our trainees with a healthy recreational outlet. We encouraged all of our new people to continue any musical interests they may have had before they lost their sight or, if possible, develop new interests in either listening to music or learning to play an instrument. I remember in 1961 we had an unusually talented group of trainees who organized a small combo to perform at events like the Sight Conservation Forum. The group included Bill Smith of Fort Smith on the saxaphone and Bobby Long on lead guitar. Smith once played with the Smith Family Band on the Grand Old Opry and Long, who studied under the famous guitarist Chet Atkins, had played for recording artists like Brenda Lee. That winter the little combo from the rehabilitation center played some of the best music heard in the entire state.

A final recreational activity at the center involved some of the trainees' interest in becoming ham radio operators. Initially I opposed the project since the radio equipment cost so much, but I went along with the idea because I thought using the radios might contribute to the development of trainees' communications skills. As events turned out, operating the transmitting equipment went beyond building basic skills.

In 1966 the blind ham operators at the center made the Christmas season memorable for Arkansas servicemen in Viet Nam and their families at home by enabling them to exchange messages across the ocean. Two years later an emergency team from the AEB provided communications at Jonesboro, in northeast Arkansas, after a tornado killed thirty-four people and destroyed large sections of the town. Finally, in 1970, when Hurricane Celia ripped through South Texas, the Red Cross declared the short-wave station at the center in Little Rock an emergency communications facility. For several days, teams of blind trainees worked on a twenty-four hour schedule to maintain communications with the devastated areas. As a result of their efforts, several lives were saved and the whole experience provided all of our trainees with a marvelous example of sighted and blind people working side by side to accomplish important goals, the kind of world we hoped they would find after completing their training and leaving the center.

We designed all of our programs — orientation and mobility, daily living techniques, communications skills and recreational activities to help instill confidence in our trainees and prepare them to function in a sighted environment. None of these activities, however, could have succeeded without the hard work and dedication of the staff members who labored over the years to provide the best possible environment for our clients.

Perhaps the most irreplaceable staff member from the beginning of the adjustment center has been Lila Lampkin. A native of Danville, Arkansas and a graduate of Draughan's Business College, Lila joined my staff as a secretary when I moved from the Welfare Department to the Education Department and worked on every step of the planning process that created the center. After I decided to join the volunteer agency as a paid employee, I knew I would need a secretary, so I invited Lila to come with me. Even though I pointed out she would be sacrificing a good deal in terms of retirement benefits, she chose to become part of the staff at the center anyway.

From the beginnning, Lila became personally involved in our work. She joined the American Association of Workers for the Blind and served as assistant secretary to the board of both the Arkansas Enterprises for the Blind and the Lions State Committee for Sight Conservation. After a few years she was promoted to the position of Administrative Assistant. From that post Lila seemed to know everything that went on at the center and anticipated a variety of needs and necessary actions. Knowing the difficulties we faced in the beginning,

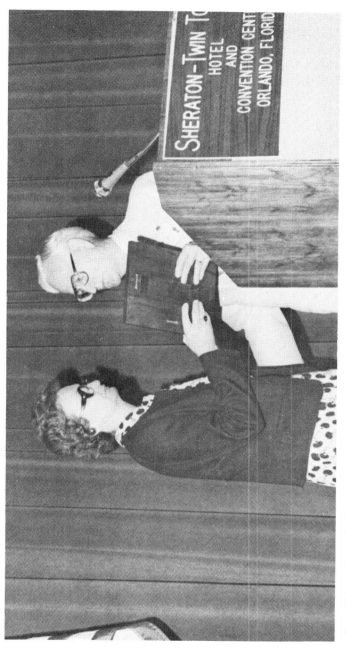

Roy Kumpe had the honor of presenting Lila Lampkin, longtime AEB secretary and administrative assistant, the Alfred Allen award at the 1982 American Association of Workers for the Blind convention in Orlando, Florida.

she also acted as a guardian against needless waste — turning off unused lights or saving supplies whenever possible. Many times I had to force her to take a long overdue vacation and when I retired in 1978, Lila remained as the admistrative assistant to the two directors that followed me. I sometimes wonder if the center would have turned out as it did without Lila's loyal and dedicated service.

Another important staff member who played a key role in the development of the center was Oliver H. Burke. Oliver had been a bookkeeper and accountant before entering the Army during World War II. Wounded by artillery fire near Aachen, Germany, he returned to the United States with a severe visual handicap. I first heard about him in the spring of 1951 when he was completing his bachelor's degree at the University of Central Arkansas (then called Arkansas State Teachers College). I recruited him to come to work at the center and personally trained him in orientation and mobility.

Oliver had never been around blind people but almost immediately became enthusiastic about our work. After a short time I made him our first full-time orientation and mobility instructor. At first I assumed he planned eventually to enter administrative or supervisory work at the center, but Oliver told me one day that he felt his most important contribution would be as a mobility teacher. He had discovered an occupation at which he excelled and wanted to continue the work he enjoyed. He stayed with us for over twenty-five years and when he retired, I would guess Oliver Burke had taught more blind people independent travel than any other person in the world.

In January, 1951 I escorted a group of trainees to the movie *Bright Victory* staring Arthur Kennedy and Peggy Dow. There is a powerful scene in the film when the recently blinded hero caresses a mirror, unwilling to admit he will never see his own reflection again. This incident vividly portrayed the severe emotional shock that accompanies blindness. For almost every newly blinded individual a period of incredible depression follows the loss of sight. Some people tell themselves their condition is only temporary — that soon some medical breakthrough or religious miracle will restore their lost vision. Others become withdrawn, silently cursing their fate and refusing to restore any semblance of a normal life. A few individuals seem to actually enjoy being dependent on others and expect those around them to be available constantly to meet the every need of the poor pitiful blind person.

From my work in the stand program I knew the psychological impact of blindness and wanted desperately to be able to meet this need in our work at the center. By coincidence, soon after I started my search for a staff psychologist, a friend of mine who worked as a rehabilitation counselor in Michigan called me and recommended a young man who had just graduated with a master's degree in guidance and counseling from the University of Michigan. My friend told me he was having a difficult time finding a job for the young man because of blindness and inexperience. The counselor asked me if I would hire Lyle Thume, the blind psychologist, on an internship basis, which I enthusiastically agreed to do.

The first three months the Michigan rehabilitation program paid us while Lyle oriented himself to our program, and after that he went on our payroll, where he remained for thirteen years. Lyle made an important contribution to our program — administering and evaluating aptitude, I.Q. and other tests, counseling with the trainees and serving as a role model of a successful blind person by doing numerous things our trainees thought were limited to sighted individuals. For example, he was the first blind person I ever encountered who knew how to water ski. One weekend Berenice and I accompanied Lyle on a skiing trip to Hot Springs where he demonstrated tremendous skill and confidence as he jumped the waves and swung in a wide arc behind the boat.

Unfortunately, he somehow missed a wave and flipped over. As a child Lyle had suffered from congenital glaucoma and had to have his eyes removed and artificial eyes inserted. When he hit the water that afternoon, the blow knocked out one of his prostheses. He had a marvelous sense of humor and when he got to shore he laughed about the accident and told us he would have to run an advertisement in The Hot Springs newspaper informing the local fishermen that if they caught a fish and cut it open and "it's still looking at you, the eye belongs to Lyle Thume."

While Lyle started our counseling program at the center, Dr. Payton Kolb continued this facet of our training and expanded the service to a high professional level. Upon his return from the Korean War, Dr. Kolb volunteered his services to the AEB as a psychiatric consultant. He visited the center every Saturday morning, talking with the trainees and advising those who had unusual emotional problems. Dr. Kolb had no special training in working with the blind but he read the limited literature that existed in those days and over the years became self-trained on the subject, often presenting papers on blindness and mental health at national psychiatric meetings.

In 1958 Dr. Kolb began meeting with our staff and expanding his time with the trainees who needed his services. He has remained a part-time staff member at the center for over twenty-five years and provided valuable insights for staff members and trainees alike. He often explained that mental illness is just like physical illness and a person can recover from emotional problems just as well as from physical ones. This concept helped all of us in dealing with some of our trainees who seemed mired forever in a deep pit of depression. I will always be grateful to Dr. Kolb for providing the important and needed dimension of psychiatric counseling for our rehabilitation center.

All of our staff members — Lila Lumpkin, Oliver Burke, Lyle Thume, Dr. Kolb, and so many others — added their personal touch to the rehabilitation center. Over the years each of these individuals made a special contribution to the development of the facility and they will always be remembered for their conscientious and devoted service.

As executive director of the center my job in this formative era centered primarily on promotion and education. Raising money took a considerable amount of time as did my efforts to sell blind people on what the center could do for them. In this regard my work resembled my earlier job with the stand program — convincing blind peple they could live useful and productive lives and letting them know how the rehabilitation center could help them reach their goals. Finally, I had to convince the rehabilitation professionals that they should invest their funds on the services offered by the center. Without their referrals our program would never have reached the thousands of blind people who eventually received the training we provided.

A secondary "selling" job that I undertook during those years involved educating the general public about blindness

94

and trying to shatter some of the persistent myths that surround the loss of sight. Far too often I heard well-meaning people say how fortunate it was that when a person lost his vision he was compensated with a corresponding improvement in his capacity to hear. These myths never cease to amaze me in the degree to which the public accepts them without ever bothering to investigate their validity.

In an effort to confront these misconceptions and to sell our program at the center, I traveled thousands of miles to speak to Lions Clubs and other civic groups throughout Arkansas and the surrounding states. Whenever possible I took Lyle Thume, Oliver Burke or one of our trainees with me to help explain our program. One of the most popular presentations was a panel discussion called "Learning to Live Without Sight" which we began in 1955 and presented to various organizations for many years thereafter.

Unquestionably the most effective method of telling our story was a series of films made at the center starting in the mid-1950s. Our first movie, entitled "Living Without Sight," was written by George S. Brewer and produced by the Lions Club. Although my debut as movie director never won acclaim in Hollywood, I thought "Living Without Sight" served the purpose well by demonstrating the nature of the program at the center, showing scenes of the Brack Home and informing the public of the important role the Lions Club played in creating the facility.

Our second color movie, "Pathways to a New Life," premiered in October, 1964 at the Sight Conservation Forum. The film showed our new building and focused on the experiences of three trainees who had benefited from their training at the center. We financed the movie by selling "Miss America" license tags in honor of Donna Axum of El Dorado, Arkansas, the 1964 Miss America.

In 1971 we released "Happiness is a State of Mind," a twenty-two-minute film on the operation and philosophy of the Arkansas Enterprises for the Blind. Under a $16,000 grant from the Jess Odom Foundation, the movie included a narration by cowboy movie star Roy Rogers. Two years after its release, "Happiness is a State of Mind" had been seen in thirty-three states and some Latin American countries by rehabili-

95

tation personnel, Lions Clubs and other civic groups as well as by hundreds of concerned individuals.

Another important instrument that has helped publicize the work of the center has been our monthly newsletter, published continuously since 1954. About a year after we started the newsletter Mrs. Elizabeth Oots of Kansas City, Missouri completed her instruction at the center and, in a brief farewell speech, made the remark that "here the foundations have been laid upon which I can build a new life." From that time on we adopted the title *New Life* for our newsletter. Each month Lions throughout the country, former trainees and other interested people received the latest issue of *New Life*, which contains articles on innovative programs at the center, personnel changes and news of the achievements of our graduates. *New Life* has been an important vehicle in publicizing the work of the center and "selling" what we believe is the finest rehabilitation program for the adult blind in the world.

Arkansas's fortunes have not always included such institutions. In 1939 the state ranked forty-eighth in its work for the blind. Twenty years later, however, Arkansas ranked near the top of the field. The rehabilitation center in Little Rock made an important contribution to this dramatic rise, as did the Arkansas School for the blind and the state's Vocational Rehabilitation Department. One important aspect of this climb involved an early effort on the part of many people to aid all of the blind citizens of the state regardless of social class or race. For example, starting in the mid-1940s, the AEB initiated a concerted effort to recruit black operators for the stand program. This campaign proved to be one of the most difficult tasks I ever attempted. Because of the racial prejudice of southern whites, blacks always had difficulty finding meaningful work, and if the black person happened to be blind, finding a job was almost impossible. After many futile efforts with public and private organizations, I convinced Dr. Lawrence Davis, the president of the state's all black college, Arkansas A M & N, to allow us to establish a stand on the school campus at Pine Bluff. On December 4, 1946 a part-time preacher named Charles Johnson became our first black stand operator. Several years later, Chris Finkbeiner of the Little Rock Packing Company allowed us to open a stand with a black operator in his plant and by the early 1950s we had four black operators in the program. Despite the southern mores of that era, whenever we had sales meetings or general gatherings of our operators, everyone sat wherever they wanted. I think in many ways white blind people were more sympathetic than their sighted counterparts to the plight of American blacks because they also had experienced discrimination.

Reluctantly, we did yield on the segregation issue in establishing a separate rehabilitation center for blind black adults. Because of my earlier success in Pine Bluff, I worked closely with the black community in that city to create a facility similar to the one in Little Rock. During an organizational meeting in the summer of 1951, Viola Lee, a retired school teacher, volunteered to donate her house to serve as an adjustment center. She became the first supervisor of the facility and we named the operation the Cowan Center in honor of her parents. We launched a fundraising drive under the auspices of the Pine Bluff Lions Club that resembled our efforts four years earlier in Little Rock. The highlight of the campaign for the Cowan Center, however, was a wonderful benefit concert by the famous composer of the "St. Louis Blues," W. C. Handy. Handy, who had lost his sight some years earlier, headed the Handy Foundation for the Blind and his generous support for our project helped establish the Cowan Center on a firm financial basis.

Even with the Cowan Center in Pine Bluff, we faced the ugly spectre of racial prejudice at our facility in Little Rock. Although we had trained a black person at the center before the city's 1957 racial controversy, during the crisis we accepted a blind woman from Guam who had a dark complexion and immediately after she began her mobility training in the neighborhood, our switchboard lit up with a rash of hate calls. "Are you trying to integrate over there?" an angry caller shouted at me. "We're not going to have Negroes in this neighborhood even if they are blind." The strangest phenomenon in the whole incident was that after I explained that the individual in question was a native of Guam and not a fellow citizen of the United States, the callers backed away from their opposition.

In the early 1960s, after the AEB board phased out the Cowan Center, I invited Anthony Celebrezze, President John Kennedy's new Secretary of Health, Education and Welfare to speak at the dedication of one of our new buildings. Celebrezze's assistant phoned me and asked if the dedication would be integrated. Although I assured him this would be the case, he felt that because of Little Rock's reputation in racial matters, an "insufficient" number of blacks in the audience would be embarrassing to the secretary. I phoned Mary Switzer, the head of the federal rehabilitation program in Washington and she had the answer. She suggested we invite instead Louis Rives, the chief of the Federal Office for the Blind, who was blind himself. "He's familiar with your program down there," Mary said, "and besides, he won't see whether it's integrated or not."

From the day we admitted our first trainee in 1947, the people associated with the adjustment center began building the foundations that sustained the program for over thirty years. Our basic services — orientation and mobility, daily living techniques, communications skills, recreational activities and psycho-social and vocational evaluations — remained the core of our services. Staff members like Lila Lampkin, Oliver Burke, Lyle Thume and Payton Kolb began a tradition of dedicated service in those early days. But the key ingredient in making our program a success was a unique group of blind people who came to the center to learn how to live a meaningful existence and build a new life. These were the individuals who bore the lion's share of making the center a special kind of place.

CHAPTER 7
The Lion's Share

In Ernesto Sabato's 1950 novel *The Outsider*, the protagonist says ". . . I must now confess that I do not like blind people at all and that in their presence I feel something of the same sensation that cold, damp and silent animals, such as snakes, give me." Unfortunately those same sentiments still too often underlie the attitude with which sighted people regard the blind. The blind are too different. They act peculiar. They only like to be around other blind people. They are somehow inferior. Over the years numerous trainees at our center have told me essentially the same story. "When I go shopping with a sighted person," they say, "sometimes the clerk gives my change to the person with me as if I don't exist."

As a matter of common sense, blind people are not that different from their sighted counterparts. People who lose their sight do not forfeit their intelligence or their imagination or their reasoning power or their sense of humor. They do not cease to be loving, friendly or courageous human beings. Most importantly, blind people are individuals. They have individual dreams, needs and potentials. One of our main goals at the AEB has been to restore a sense of dignity and selfworth to people blinded as adults. Because so much effort is expended on the reclamation of a single person, the value of the individual is a theme that dominates virtually everything we do at the center.

My most cherished hope is that more and more of the sighted community will judge blind people as individual human beings and not as a group totally separated from the mainstream of American life. I think this dream might come true if more people knew personally some of the trainees who have gone through our program at the AEB. For the most part they are wonderful people. Oftentimes their stories are studies

99

in hope and courage. A few even reach heroic proportions in the quiet dignity with which they have restructured the course of their lives.

When most of our trainees first arrive at the center they are in a stage similar to a butterfly waiting for a chance to emerge from its cocoon and we provide what we hope will be, in the words of songwriter Paul Simon, a "bridge over troubled water" to enable them to resume responsible and productive places in their respective communities.

One of the first and most outstanding individuals to cross that bridge was a young man from Nashville, Arkansas named A. B. "Bunk" Goodrum. My long association with Bunk began in the mid-1950s with a phone call from a member of the Nashville Lions Club. My Lion friend told me about a recent graduate of their local high school who had gone to Houston, Texas to work but had returned home totally blind. The Lion had no idea what had caused the young man to lose his sight. He told me that although Bunk Goodrum had been an excellent student and member of the high school football team before he went to Texas, he had now become a recluse in his family home in Nashville.

I referred the matter to the vocational rehabilitation office and they sent a counselor to talk to Bunk and his family. The counselor reported that Bunk refused to see him and closed the file with a note that the "person was not interested in rehabilitation." On a hunch, I telephoned my contact in Nashville and asked him if he thought Bunk's parents might be able to influence him to at least visit our facility in Little Rock. He informed me that Bunk's mother and father were separated and the mother had to work to put an older son through Henderson State College in Arkadelphia. I told the Lion that I understood Bunk's experience. He felt embarrassed and ashamed and I knew a personal visit from me would not change his feelings, so I encouraged my friend to try to convince Bunk's mother to bring her son to Little Rock.

A few weeks later the young man and his mother arrived at the center. At the time Bunk suffered from an intense state of depression, responding to polite inquiries with monosyllabic grunts. I escorted the two of them on a tour of our facility, explaining the nature of the program and introducing them to our staff and trainees. Mrs. Goodrum soon became convinced

Bunk needed the services we provided and that same afternoon she completed the necessary paperwork for his admission to the center.

Over the next six weeks Bunk's personality changed completely. He learned that he could be independent again, could participate in social activities and date young ladies. He discovered he did not have to live the remainder of his life as a hermit, locked away in his mother's house in Nashville. In that brief period of time his natural outgoing personality re-emerged and he became one of our most popular trainees.

He also shed his suspicions of those who wanted to help him. One afternoon when he and I were strolling around the grounds, Bunk stopped and said, "Mr. Kumpe, you know I just couldn't believe it when I first came over here and I heard those people talking and laughing. I thought it was all a setup you'd planned just to impress me."

On another occasion I stopped by Bunk's room to discuss his future. All of our tests indicated he had the capabilities of doing college work, but I suspected he might not be interested in returning to school. I asked him frankly why he hadn't attended college after he finished high school.

"I wanted to," he said. "But I knew I couldn't because my older brother already attended Henderson and I knew my mother couldn't afford to send both of us. That's why I went off on that construction job in Texas." He proceeded to tell me about waking up one morning in Houston and discovering he had lost his sight. I questioned him further and discovered he had suffered from detached retinas, a malady that often affects its victims with sudden and irreparable blindness.

Encouraged by his rapid progress at the center, I urged Bunk to consider going to college. I explained that the vocational rehabilitation laws entitled him to have all the cost of his books and tuition paid by the government. I also counseled him to attend Henderson because his brother could help him if the need arose. Before he left for school, Bunk completed a Dale Carnegie course which increased his self-confidence and I had great hopes he would do well at Henderson.

Bunk's success in college exceeded my every expectation. His classmates elected him president of the freshman class and later president of the sophomore and junior classes and vice president of the student body. Excelling in the classroom and

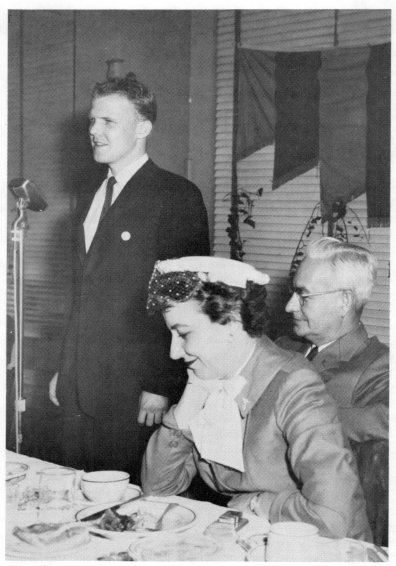

A major part of AEB's public relations effort has been trainees and staff members speaking to Lions Clubs and state Lions meetings. A. B. "Bunk" Goodrum, who fit both categories, addressed the Lions Mid-Winter Conference in Fort Smith in 1958.

in extracurricular activities, he graduated with a degree in education. Before Bunk finished his degree, the instructors at Henderson tried to convince him to do his practice teaching at the School for the Blind. The rehabilitation counselor and I traveled to Arkadelphia to attempt to dissuade them. I knew he could do the job in public school and I wanted to shatter the myth that a blind person could only teach blind children.

During the course of the meeting at the college, the young man who placed the practice teachers in various school districts became rather vexed at the whole situation and finally said, "What will the school people think about us here at Henderson if we send them a blind person?" Prejudice takes many forms and Bunk and I met his remark with a long and icy silence.

Immediately upon returning home I contacted some friends of mine at Little Rock Central High School, one of the nation's most outstanding secondary schools, and asked them if they would consider allowing Bunk to do his practice teaching there. They agreed and Bunk Goodrum became the first blind person to complete his practice teaching in a public school in Arkansas. He taught history and kept his lecture and lesson notes in braille. Excelling in the classroom, he became one of the most popular teachers on the campus that term.

After his graduation from Henderson, Bunk won a scholarship for a professional training course at the Industrial Home for the Blind in Brooklyn, New York. I was so proud of this young man. Only a few years earlier he had been afraid to even leave his own house and now he could travel alone to New York for a twenty-week training course. After Bunk completed his program in Brooklyn, I offered him a job at the center. Because of his record and his personality, he unquestionably could have worked in the public schools, but I also knew he would be a tremendous inspiration to our new trainees. He accepted my offer and joined our staff as a braille instructor. Gradually he became involved in our public relations efforts, speaking to Lions Clubs and other groups throughout the state. After a few years he took a leave of absence and earned his master's degree in guidance and counseling from the University of Arkansas.

Frankly, I harbored great expectations that someday Bunk would become the executive director of the rehabilitation center in Little Rock. However, his talents and ambitions led him in a different direction. He became a rehabilitation counselor in Houston, Texas, where, after receiving a promotion to area supervisor, he eventually became the director of rehabilitation at the Lighthouse of Houston, Texas.

When Bunk married one of our sighted home economics teachers, he asked me to serve as his best man at the wedding and I gladly accepted the honor. .Bunk Goodrum is an outstanding individual who symbolizes what blind people can accomplish when they decide to pursue their own dreams and abandon a reclusive life of self-pity. Our goal at the rehabilitation center has always been to provide people like Bunk with the necessary tools to achieve those goals — to provide a "bridge over troubled water."

While blindness is unquestionably a severe handicap, the loss of sight does not necessarily destroy an individual's talent. I cannot think of a better example of a blind person who developed a natural talent and used it to its fullest potential than a young lady from New Orleans named Candy Riedel.

Candy came to the AEB center for our college preparatory course in the summer of 1968. We had started this program seven years earlier under a research and demonstration grant from the federal government. The course served blind high school graduates who had an outstanding scholastic background. During a special nine-week summer course, the college prep students received the same instruction our regular trainees plus additional academic work and discussions dealing with various problems they might encounter as college students — how to locate readers, how to get books transcribed, the importance of extracurricular activities, how to take effective class notes. As part of the program we also had our students audit a regular college course at the University of Arkansas at Little Rock, which is located two blocks from the AEB campus.

Candy Riedel entered our college prep program with excellent credentials. After attending the Louisiana School for the Blind for a few years, she transferred to a girls' Catholic school, where she maintained an outstanding academic record. She had a fine mind and enrolled at Loyola University in New Orleans the fall after completing her training at the center.

104

The following spring Candy wrote me asking if she could return to Little Rock in the summer and work at the center as a volunteer. I accepted her generous offer and that summer Candy provided a fine addition to our staff. A music major at Loyola, she worked in our recreational program, playing the piano and leading group singing sessions. When she returned the next summer, we supplied her room and meals while she continued to expand the musical side of our recreational activities.

In July the Governor's Committee for Employment of the Handicapped met in Hot Springs and the program chairman asked me if we had any talented young people at the center. I took Candy to the meeting where she played the piano and sang for the group. I knew after that that Candy Riedel had a promising future in the field of music.

Suggesting she alter her course of study slightly and major in music therapy, I hoped that Candy might someday return to our center and develop a complete program of musical recreation. When she discussed the change with her guidance counselor at Loyola, however, he discouraged her because the internships for music therapy majors usually took place in mental hospitals and he felt that would be a dangerous situation for a blind person. Although I thought his attitude reflected a lack of understanding of both blindness and mental illness, he managed to convince Candy to continue her major in musical education.

Following her graduation, she worked at the center for a few years, but I suspected in a matter of time her ability would lead her in a different direction. One day a talent agent heard her sing at a wedding and offered her an audition at a night-club in the French Quarter in New Orleans. Candy turned down the position because she considered it inappropriate for her, but a few months later she received another job offer — as a piano bar entertainer at Dan's International Lounge in Fats' City, a section of New Orleans where neighborhood people go to avoid the tourists.

Candy accepted the spot at Dan's and has worked there for over five years, attracting a loyal local following. I've visited New Orleans several times since Candy left Little Rock and on each trip I've stopped by Dan's to hear her perform. She adds new songs and her show changes and improves each time I

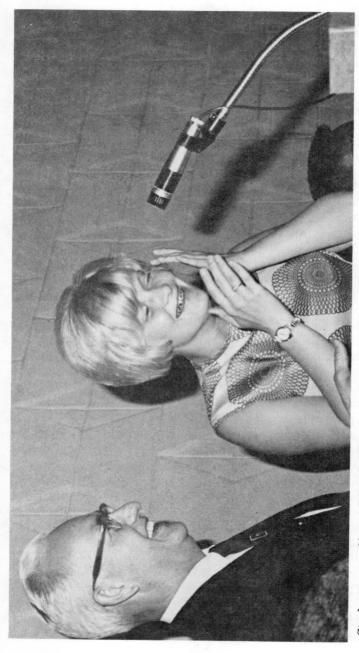

Students attending AEB's College Preparatory training vie for cash scholarships. Roy Kumpe informs Evelyn Penman of Tucson that she has won a scholarship during 1968.

hear her. One thing that does not change is the quiet pride I feel whenever I hear Candy's voice — the voice of a young blind person developing her talent to its utmost capability.

One afternoon in the early 1950s, I received a call from the director of the Services for the Blind in Oklahoma City. He informed me that he had a young man there who had recently been blinded in a gunshot accident. Through an unusual set of family circumstances the young man was about to be released from the hospital, but had no place to go. Since we had bed space available at the center, I agreed to take him as a trainee although this was the first case we had ever accepted directly from the hospital.

Jerry Dunlap had only been blind for three weeks when he came to the center in Little Rock. I vividly remember the Saturday afternoon he arrived because we were having a dance for the trainees that evening. I debated with myself whether to take Jerry to the dance since he had just joined us, but finally decided that the dance could teach him an immediate and valuable lesson — that blind people could still have fun. Although Jerry did not participate in the festivities much that night, several of our younger trainees like Bunk Goodrum stopped by and welcomed him to the center and the positive feelings from that first experience provided a solid foundation for Jerry's adjustment training.

Our new trainees had usually been blind for three or four years and had learned from their families how a blind person "should" act. In Jerry's case he had not been blind long enough to develop any bad habits and consequently adapted quickly to mobility training and the other facets of our program. Jerry became friends with Lyle Thume, our blind psychologist, and Lyle later told me that when Jerry first came to the center he had not had time to recover from the shock of his blindness and fully realize what had happened to him.

Having completed high school, Jerry had planned to attend college and study forestry at the time of his accident. We encouraged him to pursue his goal of returning to school although we also helped him investigate some alternative avenues of study. Following a four-month training period at the center, Jerry returned to his native state and entered the University of Oklahoma at Norman. Toward the end of his freshman year he wrote a note informing me he had decided to become a counselor like Lyle Thume and asking if he could spend the summer at the center to help our new trainees in exchange for his room and board. I thought the arrangement would be mutually beneficial and Jerry returned to the center that summer.

After finishing his bachelor's degree in psychology at the University of Oklahoma (and marrying the young coed who served as his reader), Jerry attended Texas Tech in Lubbock where he received his master's in psychology and counseling. Returning to Oklahoma, he started his career as a counselor in the state's rehabilitation program before becoming a supervisor, and finally program administrator of Visual Services.

While Jerry's vocational success certainly pleased me a great deal, I also applauded his active involvement in our professional organizations. He helped organize the first chapter of the American Association of Workers for the Blind in Oklahoma and served as the group's first president. In 1979, after a term on the national board of the AAWB, Jerry Dunlap became the national president of the association — the same position I had held almost thirty years earlier. As president of the AAWB, Jerry acted as a delegate to the World Council for the Welfare of the Blind which met in Antwerp, Belgium in 1979. I represented the International Services for the Blind at that same meeting and when I heard Jerry present a fine scholarly paper at the convention, I realized that he had become one of the new young leaders in the international movement to aid the blind.

During the time Jerry received his adjustment training at the center in Little Rock, he and Bunk Goodrum became close friends and I sometimes saw that relationship as a friendly sibling rivalry. Both of these men have done extremely well in their chosen careers and I regard each one of them as an example of what I had originally hoped the rehabilitation center would be able to accomplish. As I listened to the applause for Jerry Dunlp's paper in Antwerp I couldn't help but think about some of the blind people I encountered earlier in my career — those unfortunate individuals who spent most of their lives in the back bedroom or rocked their lives away in useless idleness on the front porch of a generous relative. The success of men like Bunk Goodrum and Jerry Dunlap helped demonstrate that blindness could be overcome and as Helen

Keller once said, the blind could enjoy "life's sweet accomplishments."

When we first opened the rehabilitation center in 1947, I never dreamed that someday we would be serving clients on an international basis. But after more than thirty years of operation we have trained hundreds of blind individuals from all over the world. One of the most interesting of these international trainees was a young lady from Antwerp, Belgium named Sylvia Roose. I first heard about Sylvia when I received a call from a friend of her family, a man who operated an import-export business in New York City. He told me that when Sylvia was in her mid-twenties she had been blinded in an automobile accident while vacationing in Italy. The family had searched worldwide for a rehabilitation program until the American Foundation for the Blind referred them to Little Rock.

At first the family's inclination had been to keep Sylvia at home where servants could wait on her, but she had inherited a part interest in the family printing and stationery business and wanted to learn to be independent enough to work in the office. When she first arrived in New York, several acquaintances urged her to go to the Carroll Rehabilitation Center in Boston because of its location on the east coast. Some of these people even told her she probably would not be able to understand the kind of English spoken in Arkansas. The idea that Arkansas could have a quality program on a level with those in New York or Boston or Philadelphia has always been a difficult concept for our eastern friends to accept.

After a thorough investigation Sylvia decided to stick to her original decision and participate in our course in Little Rock. She spent about six months with us, where she concentrated on typing and switchboard training along with other basic skills like mobility and personal management. I visited with her several times and discovered that her father had been a charter member of the first Lions Club in Belgium. I found it ironic that years later his daughter would benefit from a facility sponsored by Lions Clubs.

After completing her training, Sylvia returned to Belgium where, over her mother's protests, she rented her own apartment, did her own housekeeping and worked every day in the family business. A few years later she came back to Little

Rock for a refresher course in mobility and braille. During that period she revealed to me that since her brothers were doing an excellent job of managing the family business, she had decided to stay in the United States. A few months after our conversation she married one of our mobility instructors, set up housekeeping in an apartment in Little Rock and enrolled in classes at University of Arkansas at Little Rock, ready to pursue a totally new life.

One of the most courageous trainees that ever participated in our program at the center was Ann Johnston. During Ann's freshman year in medical school at the University of South Carolina, she lost her sight from diabetic retinopathy. She had been a child diabetic and had always held to a single purpose in her life — to study medicine and engage in research for the treatment of diabetes. But the disease robbed her of her sight before she could achieve that goal.

Like most victims of diabetic retinopathy, Ann went blind suddenly and found herself in a wake of emotional trauma and depression. After several months a rehabilitation counselor in South Carolina referred her to our center for adjustment and prevocational training. She wanted to enter our new program to prepare to become a taxpayer service representative. Her father worked for the Internal Revenue Service and knew about our success in teaching blind people to act as liaisons between the IRS and the public.

For Ann's part, the reorganization of her life's goals from medicine to a career in the Internal Revenue Service posed serious problems. From her first day at the center, however, Ann Johnston demonstrated a rare combination of courage and determination. She went through all the steps of psychological, social and vocational adjustment. She learned mobility, new communications skills and daily living techniques and, after only four months, passed the difficult evaluation test for the IRS program.

While undergoing her adjustment training, Ann also became an active member of the community. She sang in the choir of a nearby Baptist church, joined several local organizations and interacted with sighted people on a regular basis.

Ann's TSR class in Little Rock included a nice young man from Boston and about a year after she left to become a service representative in her home state of South Carolina, I received a wedding announcement. Since they had met while participating in our program, Ann and her husband returned to Arkansas for their honeymoon. A few months later they moved to Boston, where she resumed her work for the IRS while her husband pursued a career in the state Attorney General's office.

Some time later I received a letter from Ann telling me about her recent promotion to training supervisor. In that capacity she instructed sighted people in the intricacies of the laws and codes that govern our system of taxation. Through her own resolution and enterprise, with a little guidance from the center, Ann Johnston reorganized her life and demonstrated that blind people are perfectly capable of being productive citizens.

Our theme at the AEB has always been to help blind adults find a "new life." Billie Elder's experience with our program illustrates what can be accomplished when a blind person resolves to achieve that goal. When Mrs. Elder first arrived at the center in 1964, her life had reached a low point. A middle-aged wife and mother, she had gradually lost her sight from a disease called retinitis pigmentosa. In the immediate aftermath of her blindness, her Methodist minister husband became ill and had to be hospitalized in their home town in Tennessee for an extended period of time.

Mrs. Elder's indomitable spirit carried her through our adjustment program. Because she had been a teacher before the onset of blindness, at the conclusion of her training I asked her to remain at the center as a braille instructor. In that capacity she was not only an excellent teacher but also served as an inspiration to our new trainees. After a while she became interested in our overall program and took a leave of absence to study for her master's degree in rehabilitation teaching at Western Michigan University.

When she returned to Little Rock, I named her the Supervisor of Educational Services at the AEB. As her interest in the cause of the blind grew, Mrs. Elder became active in the American Association of Workers for the Blind and in 1975 she was elected vice president of the American Council of the Blind.

One of Billie Elder's favorite sayings is that "when life caves in, you are either buried or planted." Through her own

111

inner strength Mrs. Elder took charge of her own survival and, with the help of our staff and the Tennessee Rehabilitation Services, carved a new life for herself: a life filled with new experiences and opportunities for growth — a chance to be planted rather than buried.

Sometimes a "new life" can simply be the independence to return to the activities and routines of an "old life." I recall a series of conversations on the porch at the center with a trainee named Betty Miller, that illustrated to me that a "new" life does not always have to be new. The mother of three children from suburban Tulsa, Oklahoma, Betty had suffered from "night blindness" for several years, but dismissed her condition as a common problem for adults.

Then, on Christmas Day, 1966 her visual problem became acute. Looking at the twinkling lights on the family Christmas tree, she realized all the colors had blurred together. Covering her right eye, she discovered that out of her left eye she could see only an image about the size of a dinner plate.

Her sight continued to deteriorate and after years of frustrating visits to various doctors, an eye specialist in Massachusetts finally correctly diagnosed her problem. Betty had retinitis pigmentosa, a hereditary disease which causes a gradual degeneration of the retina. The disease left Betty without any sight in her left eye and with minimal light perception in her right eye.

Initially, Betty tried to continue her regular activities such as a weekly trip to a cross town shopping mall and volunteer work at her local church. But following a series of embarrassing incidents the outings ceased after about a year. Once, she got into a police car, mistaking the vehicle for a taxi cab and on another occasion, while trying to walk to church she took a wrong turn and became lost in a neighbor's backyard.

"That was when I began sitting in the house," she told me later. "I was too frightened to go out. I became depressed and anxious and wondered what the future held for me and if it was all worth it."

Working through counselors at the Oklahoma Division of Visual Services, Betty and her husband Dave, a public relations executive, arranged for her to enter the AEB center in Little Rock. A couple of days after she arrived we had our first chat on the sunny "solar porch" on the center's multi-purpose building. "You can go from doctor to doctor and chase butter-flies and rainbows," she said then, "but there is a time when you finally have to sit down and face it. I knew I would either have to come here or stay home and become a vegetable."

After a short time, Betty became one of our most enthusi-astic trainees. "The two weeks I've been here have given me more confidence than I had in my entire life," she told me at a second meeting. "I feel that if I want to go to the snack bar and get a cup of coffee, I can do it even if I can't see the way!"

She went through our basic program with the goal of re-turning to Tulsa and resuming her duties as a wife and mother. Six months later she did just that. I spoke with her briefly the morning she left for home and her changed outlook on her condition made me realize that being able to return to her former existence constituted a "new life" for Betty Miller. "I don't want to be treated like a cripple and babied and hovered over," she said. "I'll ask for help when I need it. Otherwise, I'll do things on my own. I'm not going to sit in the house alone ever again."

The two most unusual trainees that ever participated in our program were a Korean War veteran and a stout lady from the hill country. I first heard about the former soldier through a frantic phone call from the state director of rehabilitation in Texas. He said he had a young man named Archie McKnight* who had not only been blinded in the war, but had received enough other injuries to qualify for a hundred percent dis-ability. As a result, he received a fairly large check from the government every month.

Unfortunately, McKnight squandered his money on alcohol and women and the Veterans Administration had given up on him as a hopeless case. The rehabilitation director thought participation in a program like ours might restore a young veteran's confidence and stability and asked if I would be willing to accept him. Since I wanted to cultivate a relation-ship with the Texas rehabilitation counselors, I reluctantly agreed.

We always admitted new trainees on Monday in order to take advantage of a full staff. However, the counselor from Texas brought Archie to Little Rock on Saturday afternoon. When I arrived at the office on Monday morning, the young

*Not his real name.

lady who had admitted Archie informed me he had brought a gun with him. He had checked the pistol with his other valuables at the desk, and when I asked him about the weapon he said it was a souvenir of his experience in Korea. Even at the time I thought the fact that he brought two boxes of cartridges for his souvenir a bit unusual.

Over the course of the next two weeks, Archie McKnight antagonized everyone at the center. Because of his war record, he had an insufferable sense of superiority to other blind people and openly treated our staff with contempt. He also developed a crush on one of our female clients who was dating another young male trainee. Archie and the girl's boyfriend exchanged harsh words on several occasions.

One afternoon, in the midst of a staff meeting, one of our secretaries quietly slipped into the room and informed me Archie had appeared at the front desk, announced he wanted to leave and requested his valuables. "You didn't give him the gun, did you?" I asked, almost afraid to hear the answer.

"Yes sir, I did," the secretary said. "You told me to always give the trainees their things when they leave."

I rushed to the outside door where I found Archie wandering around the side of the building. "Where are you going, Archie?" I asked from the door. He didn't answer. One of the sighted instructors informed me the young veteran had the gun in his hand. Fearing Archie wanted to challenge the girl's boyfriend, I told a member of the staff to circle around the building and lock the doors from the inside to protect the trainees.

By the time Archie reached the entrance to the room where the other trainees were enjoying a special program, the staff member had managed to lock the door. Archie stood outside, pounding on the door and shouting the name of his rival over and over in an ominous chant. After phoning the police, I moved into the courtyard to try and dissuade the veteran from his mission.

Then the gun went off. I immediately pressed my back against the wall, fearing that Archie wanted to shoot me. After a few agonizing minutes that seemed like an eternity, two police cars whipped into the parking lot. I cautioned the officers that while Archie was blind, he was still an ex-soldier who knew how to use the gun.

114

With admirable courage, two of the policemen finally convinced Archie to drop his weapon. When one of the officers grabbed him, however, Archie put up a terrible struggle that only ended when all four policemen dragged him to the patrol car.

Later that day I learned how close to tragedy we had come. A bullet from Archie's gun had passed through the door into the room where Sam Wilkes, one of our instructors, had been trying to herd the trainees out the back way. The bullet had ricocheted off the tile floor and hit the ceiling, knocking plaster over Sam's leg.

I learned several important lessons from the incident, including never to accept a client without a full medical history. We also changed our policy to require a careful check for guns, knives or other weapons whenever a trainee first arrived.

Unfortunately, we could not help every blind person referred to the AEB. Archie's war experiences had left permanent emotional scars that we could never overcome. Consequently, our whole staff tried to put the incident behind us as quickly as possible and turn our attention to the many trainees we could assist.

One of those trainees we felt we could help was a stout woman named Mary. After Mary had been at the center for a short time she fell on the stairs and injured her leg. About a week later, Ms. Rena Metcalfe, our supervisor, phoned me at two o'clock in the morning to report that Mary had terrible abdominal pains and had screamed and cried all night. I phoned a doctor who lived near the center and who had helped us during previous emergencies. He diagnosed Mary's ailment as an acute appendicitis and gave her something for the pain, planning to remove her to the hospital later that morning.

At 7 a.m. Ms. Metcalfe phoned me again to tell me Mary's roommate thought Mary had a baby in their room. I told Ms. Metcalfe I would hold the phone while she investigated the matter. When she returned a few minutes later she breathlessly informed me that "Oh yes, Mary does have a baby in the room!"

"You call the ambulance," I said. "And I'll call the hospital."

The rehabilitation people in Mary's home state, the doctor who administered an admission physical and the physician who treated her at 2 a.m. had all failed to diagnose Mary's pregnancy. After the doctor left that morning, Mary had delivered the baby herself, walked across the hall and wrapped the infant in some towels she found in a linen closet.

Of course, we immediatley sent both Mary and her baby to the hospital and phoned the child welfare department. Mary swore she did not know about her condition and had no idea who had fathered the child. Eventually, Mary consented to give the baby up for adoption. Her roommate later confided in me she thought the baby resulted from a single incident when a young man took advantage of Mary while she was intoxicated.

I explained to Mary that we did not want to make any moral judgments in the matter and assured her we would welcome her back at the center. She returned home for almost a year and then resumed her training in Little Rock. After completing her program she married and later gave birth to four more children.

Through the years we have trained over five thousand blind adults at the AEB in Little Rock. Many of these trainees represented a story of personal courage and accomplishment. For example, Med Donaldson of Paragould, Arkansas at the age of eighty-four became the oldest trainee we ever served. Med's colorful career included service in the Spanish-American War, a tour as a trick rider with a Wild West show, four years as one of Arkansas's original game wardens and several years as a state policeman. A fiercely independent man, Med came to us to learn to get around downtown Paragould by himself and learn enough braille to read the titles on the talking books he received in the mail. Even at eighty-four, Med Donaldson refused to allow blindness to prevent him from establishing a new life.

Of course, we served thousands of other trainees whose stories were no less dramatic: Charles B. Edwards from Conway, Arkansas, who following his training, returned to his chosen occupation as an insurance agent and received the company's nationwide "agent of the year" award; Reverend Richard Ludden, a Methodist minister from Indianapolis who thought his ministering days had ended when he lost his sight, but instead became the chaplain of the AEB and for many

116

years conducted an important ministry to the blind. Finally, a thirty-six-year-old mother of three children from Houston once yielded to the pressures of a divorce and a career crisis by placing a loaded .38 caliber pistol to her temple and pulling the trigger. "After I shot myself," she told me later, "I never lost consciousness. It was like God and I were having a battle and God said I would live." The gunshot left her blind in both eyes, and I have rarely encountered a more despondent individual. After months of training and therapy, however, the young woman gained a new and more positive outlook. She became a medical transcriptionist and began doing independent counseling with both blind and sighted individuals who, like herself, had temporarily lost their way. Her new life, then, became an important instrument in helping others find their own fresh start.

Blind people are individuals. They have individual hopes and dreams and fears. Some cope with their blindness better than others, while some never even try to re-establish a normal existence. In over thirty years of working with the rehabilitation center I have met all kinds of blind people. Some of them have been the most remarkable individuals I've ever encountered. People like Bunk Goodrum, Jerry Dunlap, Ann Johnston and so many others have, with hard work and quiet dignity, molded a new life for themselves. I only wish the central character of Sabato's *The Outsider* could have met some of these remarkable people.

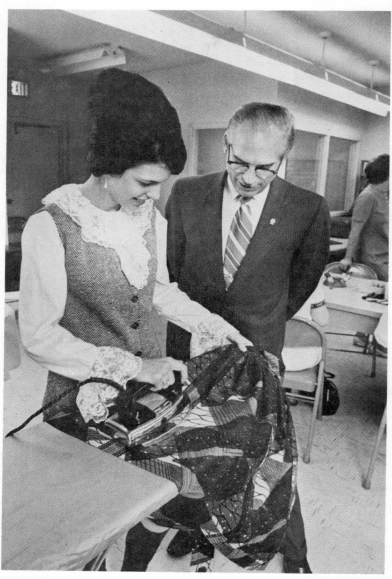

Dr. Robert McCullough of Tulsa, Oklahoma, the 50th president of Lions International and a visitor during the 1970 Visiting District Governor Day, served a term on AEB's board of directors. Here he watches a blind trainee iron a dress.

118

CHAPTER 8

The AEB in the Age of Aquarius

For many years the Little Rock Lions Club sponsored an annual stag party and at each function some of our members enjoyed organizing a low stakes crap game. Dr. Guy Smith, a blind chiropractor and one of my oldest and closest friends in the club, loved to shoot craps and enthusiastically participated in the game each year. Of course, whenever he threw the dice, one of the sighted members had to tell him the results.

One night upon receiving the dice, Guy dropped them in his pocket and rolled with a pair of brailled dice. Touching the dice at the end of the table, he hollered "seven" and began to collect everyone's money.

Several players began grumbling and one even said, "Hey Guy, how do we know that's a seven?"

Guy laughed and replied, "I've been trusting you for years. Why can't you trust me one time?"

I always thought Guy made a more serious point that evening than he intended. Trust is an important element in the relationship between the blind and the sighted community and to a large extent, blind people have to trust their sighted friends to assist them in achieving their individual goals. One of the best examples to illustrate this point is the assistance received by the AEB from so many good friends in our efforts to expand our facilities and programs to enable blind people to become responsible and productive citizens.

We conducted our first major capital funds campaign in 1959 for the purpose of constructing four new buildings on our property at Fair Park and Tyler Streets. We had outgrown the Brack Home and although we only had twenty-two clients, I believed that in the near future we would need to serve as many as fifty trainees at a time. After contacting the architectural firm of Swaim and Allen, I also convinced our board to hire a landscape architect because I wanted our new site to be attractive.

Traditionally schools and workshops for the blind have rarely been aesthetically pleasing places and have often been described as depressing. In fact, architects even designed some of the first schools for the blind without windows because they assumed blind people would not need any light. Determined that our new facility would run counter to this trend I wanted an inviting and cheerful place for our future trainees.

We encountered our first obstacle in this regard when the landscape architect informed me he thought crowding the proposed buildings on our two-thirds block property would be a mistake. To resolve the problem I approached our neighbors who owned the remainder of the block and convinced them to sell us their land. This acquisition proved extremely important because we were able to arrange our new buildings so they faced into a spacious center quadrangle with ample open areas on the outside. This arrangement could never have been achieved without utilizing the entire block.

Unquestionably our biggest hurdles in creating the new complex related to the funding of the project. After careful study of various laws in this area, I concluded that our best hope lay in seeking federal assistance through the Hill-Burton Act, a post-World War II measure to facilitate hospital construction. The act had been amended to include medical rehabilitation facilities, including some for special disabilities. Under this act the Arkansas State Health Department administered the fund and we submitted the proposal for a federal grant. The law provided for a two-thirds matching system, and with that incentive, the 1959 state Lions convention passed a resolution to raise the needed $150,000 to build the new rehabilitation facility.

Jess Odom, a prominent Little Rock insurance executive, headed our statewide fundraising campaign and Ed Barry acted as our vice chairman. At Ed's insistence we hired a professional fundraiser from Dallas named Jack McDowell. I called him "Jack the Raiser" because every time I thought we had received a generous pledge from a wealthy individual, Jack would go back and talk to the person and solicit an additional $500 or more.

120

Frankly, I did not play a major role in the solicitation part of the campaign. I believed my main function was to educate the public on the needs of the blind and I felt a little uncomfortable in asking people for money they might assume would be used to pay my salary. Throughout the drive I remained in the background, content to be involved in the detailed planning of the new facility.

I did, however, originate the Order of the Silver Cane, one of our most successful fundraising ideas. Every individual who donated $500 or more to the campaign became a member of the Order and had their name inscribed on a permanent plaque in the lobby of the new administration building. After generating several thousand dollars for our first capital funds drive, the Order of the Silver Cane remained an important part of our fundraising program.

Our overall effort raised slightly over $200,000 which, combined with the Hill-Burton money, enabled the AEB to construct the needed buildings — a men's dormitory and a women's dormitory, a new administration building that fronted on Fair Park Boulevard and a multi-purpose structure to house our training and recreational facilities. In 1961 we held a formal dedication ceremony for this new physical plant. The highlight of that function was an address by Finis Davis, the president of Lions International. What made that day so meaningful to me was the fact that in 1947, at our first dedication, one of the speeches had been delivered by the president of the Little Rock Lions Club — the same Finis Davis.

Beginning with our first capital funds campaign and extending to our expansions throughout the 1960s and 1970s, three individuals played key roles in the physical growth of the rehabilitation center — Jess Odom, Robert Sakon and Grace Pinkerton. We named our new administration facility the Jess Odom Building in honor of the man who headed our statewide campaign. During the drive Jess also personally pledged $50,000 toward the construction of the new center. Originally a businessman from Marianna, Arkansas, Jess became a self-made millionaire by organizing a series of insurance companies throughout the nation. Over the years as Lions District Governor and a member of the AEB board, Jess maintained an active interest in our program and emerged as one of

121

the center's most generous benefactors in terms of both time and money.

Our honor roll of important patrons of the AEB also includes England, Arkansas businessman Robert Sakon. Back in the early 1960s we sent Bunk Goodrum, who was then one of our staff members, to present a program on the center to the England Lions Club. Mr. Sakon liked the presentation and was impressed with the success of this blind instructor who had finished our program and had later earned a college degree. At the conclusion of the evening Mr. Sakon asked Bunk if there was any special item we wanted for the center. Bunk candidly told him that we desperately needed a new open reel tape recorder.

Mr. Sakon generously agreed to purchase the machine for us and after we acquired the recorder, I invited him to come to Little Rock to see how the new piece of equipment helped our trainees. During his visit I told him about the Order of the Silver Cane, and showed him the plaque in the foyer of the administration building. I good-naturedly said that if the recorder, which cost $300, had cost $500, he would have automatically become a member of the Order of the Silver Cane. He laughed and told me how much he admired the program at the center. Then he proceeded to write a check qualifying him for membership in the order.

Mr. Sakon's interest in the center grew and some time later he was elected to the AEB board. He believed in sharing his money while he was alive in order to see the positive things his wealth could achieve and toward the end of the decade he gave the center $21,000 to help with the cost of a fifth building in our complex.

On Sunday, June 15, 1969 we dedicated the Robert Sakon Building — a magnificent three-story structure that housed a work evaluation area, living quarters, a spacious dining room and a kitchen. Our pincipal speaker that day, Dr. Douglas MacFarland, the Chief of Services for the Blind of the Department of Health, Education and Welfare, delivered an inspirational address which served as a capstone for a decade of tremendous expansion by the AEB.

Mrs. Grace Pinkerton, a former trainee from Liberal, Missouri, provided an important foundation for that era of growth. After losing her sight from glaucoma and suffering through eight painful operations, Mrs. Pinkerton entered the AEB when she was well into her sixties. Generally, in the early years of the AEB few people over the age of forty were referred to the center, but from the beginning Grace Pinkerton proved to be a special case. For many years she had served as a distinguished nurse at a hospital in Kansas City and both the Kansas City Nursing Association and the Missouri Medical Society urged the state rehabilitation agency to refer her to our program.

A tenacious lady, Mrs. Pinkerton successfully completed her adjustment training at the center and a few months after she left Little Rock she sent us a $65 donation. In an accompanying letter Mrs. Pinkerton explained she had earned the money by selling an article about the Lions work for the blind in Arkansas to a journal called *Nursing Outlook*.

Mrs. Pinkerton maintained her interest in the AEB and a few years later contributed over $1,000 for the purchase of some ham radio equipment and over $3,000 to help pay for a van to provide our trainees with readily available transportation. Finally, in 1969, at the age of seventy-seven, Mrs. Pinkerton established a trust for the Arkansas Enterprises for the Blind which totaled over $60,000. In recognition of her philanthropy we named the women's dormitory Grace Noyes Pinkerton Hall. Pinkerton Hall has provided a genuine inspiration to our incoming trainees when we explain to them that the dormitory is named after a former trainee who built the foundations for her own new life at the AEB.

During the 1960s we did not limit the expansion of our physical plant to the construction of new buildings. In 1966 we purchased a private residence at 5321 W. 29th Street, diagonally opposite the southeast corner of our new complex. By converting the home into a housekeeping cottage for six female trainees, we expanded the center's capacity and provided a comprehensive housekeeping program for the women who expected to resume their roles as homemakers after leaving the center.

By the end of the decade the men's dormitory and the main training building remained unnamed, so I suggested to our board that the training facility on Tyler Street should be named for Ed Barry because of his leadership in the early days of the center and his years of devoted service both to the AEB

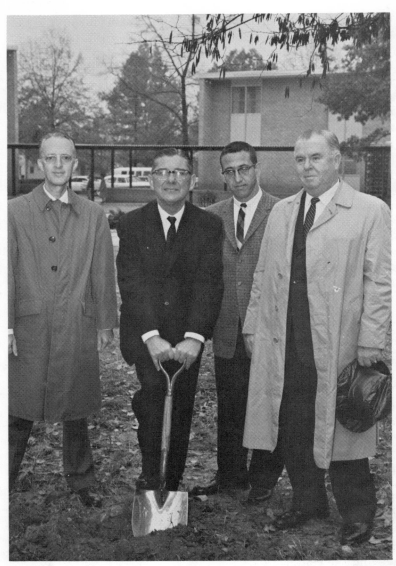

A groundbreaking ceremony for Pinkerton Hall was held in 1962. From left, Dr. J. P. Herron, state health department; U. S. Representative Wilbur D. Mills, Stanley Price of Little Rock, then president of AEB; and Edward G. Barry, Sr., the 41st president of Lions International, took part in the event.

124

and Lions International. Because of a previous out-of-town commitment I missed the next board meeting when the question would be considered. Upon my return, board president Jess Odom informed me that the members of the board had accepted my recommendation and voted to name the training building for Ed. Jess also told me that the board felt that my years of service to the AEB deserved equal recognition and had voted to name the men's dormitory Kumpe Hall.

By 1974 the AEB's annual operating budget exceeded $1,000,000 and the center employed over ninety professional and support staff. While we certainly had come a long way from our beginning in 1947, I recognized that unless we continued to expand we would soon outgrow our facility. I urged the board to explore the possibility of securing another grant under the Hill-Burton Act for the construction of some additions to our building complex.

I proposed a million-dollar campaign drive to raise the necessary matching money to build three new buildings, and Dr. Jim Fowler, a local dentist and our new board chairman, enthusiastically embraced my idea. During the installation ceremonies for the new board officers in June, 1974, Dr. Fowler challenged the board and the Lions in general to undertake the million-dollar expansion program.

My relationship with Jim Fowler went back to 1967 when, as Lions District Governor, I appointed him to the position of Zone Chairman. He was a past president of the Little Rock Founders Club and bcame a conscientious member of my cabinet. An ambitious man, Jim rose quickly through the ranks of Lionism, serving as District Governor, an international board member and eventually the Third Vice President of Lions International. When Jim became the president of the organization in 1983, he was the fourth man who started his Lions career in our state to be elected to that high office — an unusual honor for a small state like Arkansas. The other presidents with Arkansas backgrounds were Ed Barry, Finis Davis and Earl Hodges. Jim's career in the Lions movement, of course, received a strong boost from the outstanding job he did as the chairman of our Million-Dollar Expansion Fund Campaign.

We needed the money from the expansion drive to implement a three-phase building program. The first phase called for the construction of a three-level, 15,000-square-foot building to be located on the northeast corner of the campus. This facility would connect the training building and the women's dormitory and feature an enlarged physical conditioning area, a snack bar, office space for our psycho-social services, a mobility office and a library. I also wanted to include two light housekeeping apartments and two private bedrooms as part of our home management training.

The three-phase plan offered a tremendous fundraising challenge, especially in light of inflation and increased building costs. Between 1969, when we completed the Sakon Building, and 1974, when the Million-Dollar Campaign began, construction expenses had almost doubled. The matching funds requirement under the Hill-Burton Act had also changed. Instead of two-for-one matching, the revised system called for one-for-two matching. The new provisions did stipulate that the government could loan an additional one third. In other words, we had to raise one-third of the money ourselves, the second third would be covered under the grant and last third would be borrowed at three percent interest over an extended period of time.

Because of the ambitious nature of the Million-Dollar Campaign, we turned to a funding source that the AEB had never used before. During a visit to a Lions Club project in Alabama, Dr. Fowler noticed that the Lions in that state sought financial aid from the legislature and during his stay, the governor presented the Alabama Lions with a check for $250,000 in state funds. When Dr. Fowler returned to Arkansas, he launched a campaign to acquire the same kind of legislative support for our program in Arkansas. A former state senator, he discussed the matter with his numerous friends in the Senate and eventually Senator Max Howell of Jacksonville drew up a bill and agreed to sponsor the proposed legislation.

In the meantime we met with Governor David Pryor and explained our program and what we hoped to accomplish with our expansion campaign. Governor Pryor liked the project and agreed to sign the bill as soon as the measure cleared the legislature. In April, 1975 the governor signed into law Act 172 of the Arkansas legislature, appropriating a quarter of a million dollars in matching funds for the AEB's million-dollar expansion program. This act was the only time we ever asked the legislature for an appropriation.

One sidelight of our experience with Act 172 was that Governor Pryor became interested in the center. He participated in our ground-breaking ceremonies and delivered a speech to our trainees at one of their monthly banquets. The people of Arkansas later elected Governor Pryor to the United States Senate, where he has continued his interest in our work by serving as a board member and by helping us with a variety of legislative concerns. His efforts on our behalf have been matched by Arkansas' senior United States Senator, Dale Bumpers, whose interest included serving a term on our board of directors.

On April 3, 1977 the Arkansas Enterprises for the Blind formally dedicated the Dr. J.M. Fowler Building, finishing the first phase of our million-dollar expansion campaign. At my invitation, Candy Riedel returned to Little Rock to entertain our guests at the dedication ceremony and Joe Purcell, the lieutenant governor of Arkansas, delivered the major address.

The Fowler Building marked the completion of our central complex — six buildings in a square with four of them joined together in a U-shaped configuration with the administration building at the top of the U on Fair Park Boulevard. To the people who have been a part of our program since its inception in 1947 each one of those buildings represented much more than structure of brick and mortar. Each one symbolized the service and sacrifice of the individuals whose names denote each building — Jess Odom, Robert Sakon, Grace Noyes Pinkerton, Dr. Jim Fowler, Ed Barry and gratefully Roy Kumpe.

One of the nicest surprises that resulted from these capital fund campaigns was the inadvertent acquisition of a trademark for the AEB rehabilitation center. As a consequence of the publicity generated by the fundraising effort, Mrs. Winnie B. Auten phoned a member of the Pulaski Heights Lions Club and asked if our new complex on Fair Park could use a large statue of a lion.

The Lions Club member contacted Byrl A. Byles, one of our board members, and Byrl in turn asked me if I thought we could utilize the statue. My first reaction was "what in the world would we do with it?" My vision of the new complex con-

127

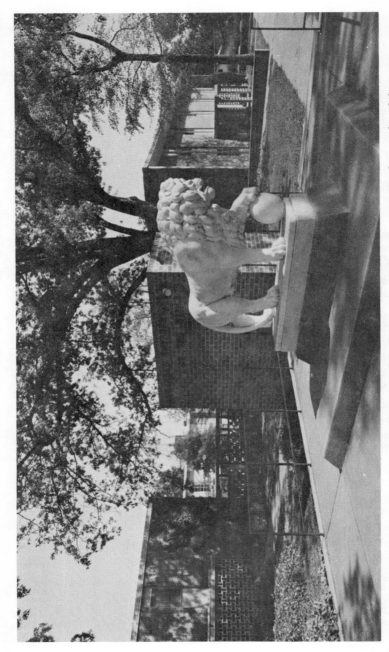

AEB campus following the initial building campaign begun in 1960 and completed in 1963.

sisted of a tight functional set of buildings with few frills and I could not see where an oversized concrete lion would fit into such a scheme. On the other hand, Mrs. Auten had aroused my curiosity, so I suggested we go look at the statue.

Mrs. Auten lived on the old Conway Highway north of Little Rock and when we arrived, Byrl and I found the lion sitting sadly beneath a large magnolia tree — stains and bird droppings covered the once proud beast and high grass and weeds camouflaged the sculpture. Mrs. Auten explained to us that their father-in-law, the late H. F. Auten, a local real estate and insurance executive, had originally purchased the lion in Italy in 1920. As she told us the history of the statue and pointed out that the sculptor had created the lion from fine Italian marble, I realized what a genuine piece of art she was offering us and what a wonderful addition the lion would make to our new complex.

Byrl felt the same way and said, "Pearl and I haven't paid our pledge to the campaign, so we'll take this lion as our personal project."

I never knew how much they paid for the statue, but he had the three-thousand-pound lion moved to the center and had the stains sandblasted away until the animal sparkled in its original white marble. We worked with our landscape architect to find the best location for the statue and he recommended we place the lion on the corner facing Fair Park with a small fountain in the background.

The AEB board finally authorized spending an additional $4,500 for the statue's location. When the members voted for the funding, I was in El Salvador helping that nation's program for the blind. My absence turned out to be a good thing because had I been in Little Rock, I am sure that my parsimonious nature would have opposed spending so much money on the project. As events turned out, the marble lion became one of the best investments in the history of the AEB. In a relatively short time that lion became the unofficial trademark of the rehabilitation center.

While many citizens of Little Rock probably have no idea exactly what goes on at the center, most of them know where the marble lion is located. That fact became clear to me the first time I met Arkansas Governor Winthrop Rockefeller. A mutual friend introduced us at a downtown Chamber of

Commerce meeting and I invited the governor to visit the AEB and see how our program operated.

At first, the governor mumbled a vague acceptance. Then his face lit up and he said, "Oh sure, you mean out there where that magnificent marble lion is — out by the university. I've always wanted to see what kind of rehabilitation program you have out there."

Every institution should have an emblem or a trademark and we were lucky to have found ours in the marble lion — a fitting symbol of both the involvement of the Lions Club and the courage of the trainees who begin their new lives at the AEB.

Since 1947, when we first opened our doors, we have tried to cultivate a good relationship with our neighbors in Oak Forest. By and large I would give our organization excellent marks in this area, although unfortunately, a few residents have resisted our expansion at every turn. Before each of our building programs began, I personally went door-to-door along both Fair Park and Tyler Streets and explained to the people who lived in the neighborhood exactly what our plans were and what our new buildings would look like.

Almost all of the residents expressed encouragement and enthusiasm for our expansion plans. However, a few (usually the same few) accused us of trying to devalue property rights and frighten property owners. Overall, after thirty years of operation, the AEB has been a good neighbor to Oak Forest and conversley the residents of Oak Forest have been good friends to the AEB.

Many of those same neighbors have actively supported our fundraising efforts by purchasing items or tickets during various campaigns. Along with annual events like the light bulb sale, the Lions Club also sponsored a variety of special events to generate money for the AEB. For example, in 1963, Governor Orval Faubus issued a special proclamation designating November 9 as Arkansas Lions Day. Lions from throughout the state gathered in Little Rock for several activities including the Lions Bowl football game between the University of Arkansas Freshmen and the University of Wichita Freshmen. The Lions donated the proceeds of the event, over $10,000, to the AEB for our general fund.

In 1975 the Lions sponsored another football game — the Bicentennial Bowl, matching Henderson State, the Arkansas small college champion against East Central Oklahoma State, the champions of Oklahoma's small college conference. Again the Lions contributed the funds raised from the event to the AEB. On that occasion the money went into the million-dollar expansion campaign and helped finance our building program.

Three years before the Bicentennial Bowl, we had another successful fundraising activity centered around a sports theme. The AEB received the gate receipts from the Lions Charity Golf Exhibition at Hot Springs Village. The match included some of the biggest stars in the Professional Golfers Association tour — Lee Trevino, Miller Barber, Dutch Harrison and Pete Fleming. Over 2,500 spectators purchased $5 tickets to see these stars perform and help the rehabilitation center at the same time.

Not all of our fund raising efforts have been statewide affairs featuring celebrities or sports events. Over the years, local Lions Clubs throughout the state have supported a variety of activities in their communities to raise money for the center. From all over Arkansas I recall dozens of pancake suppers, spaghetti suppers, Halloween candy sales, radio auctions, gospel singing events, broom sales, white cane days, turkey shoots, raffles and even an annual rabies clinic. The Lions of Arkansas donated thousands of hours to these undertakings and without their support the center would never have been able to grow as it has over the past quarter of a century.

Recently, our efforts to raise money for the AEB have centered on long-range giving. Since 1958 we have maintained sustaining memberships in the Arkansas Enterprises for the Blind, but since the mid-1970s we have put greater emphasis on donations to the center through bequests, memorials, trusts, gifts of stock, life insurance and contributions to support fellowships.

Working with Stanley Price, who has donated his legal services to the AEB for many years, the board established an endowment trust fund in 1976 to receive bequests. Soon afterward, Josephine Collie, a retired public school teacher willed the AEB a 200-acre tract of land. Lawson Glover, an attorney and past president of the AEB Board, then administered the

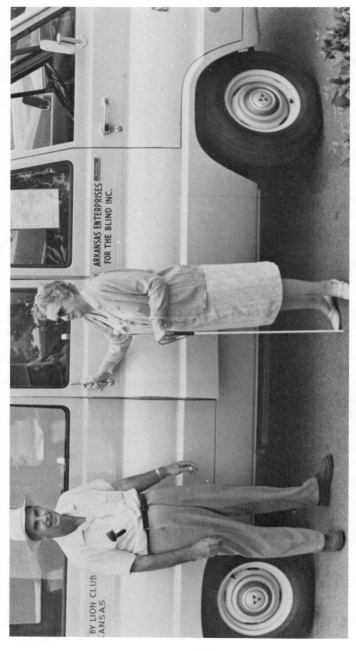

Oliver Burk, a mobility instructor at AEB for 24 years until retiring in 1975, and Mrs. Grace Pinkerton, a former trainee, stand beside the mobility travel van Mrs. Pinkerton purchased for AEB in 1969.

sale of the property for $200,000, giving our endowment fund a strong financial base. Hopefully, this type of fundraising will give the center a solid foundation not only to support existing programs but to aid in undertaking exciting new projects in the future.

The AEB has succeeded over the years as a result of its basic structure as a private nonprofit organization under the sponsorship of the Lions Club that cooperates with the federal government and the various state agencies. During the late 1960s, under the administration of President Lyndon Johnson, the federal government spent massive amounts of money on rehabilitation centers for the blind. Many of these new facilities were strictly state-operated agencies and even at the time I had misgivings about some of these enterprises. But the availability of so much money and the temptation to spend those funds proved irresistable. Regrettably, several states wound up with their own fully equipped and fully staffed programs but an insufficient blind population to justify the existence of their centers.

In one state, a center cost over five million dollars and is one of the finest state facilities in the nation. This center, however, became over-staffed, and by the late 1970s the facility spent four times per trainee what it cost the AEB in Little Rock. To make matters worse, this inefficiency has finally threatened the program to the point that some local staff members have inquired if we might be able to take over the training of some of their clients.

The unique AEB concept has been copied by several facilities in the United States and throughout the world. The idea of training the whole person rather than stressing only vocational rehabilitation has proven successful, as have our efforts to combine the resources of state and federal agencies with local civic clubs to help blind people help themselves. In an age of increasing frustration with bureaucratic red tape and inefficiency associated with state-run programs, I would proudly offer the AEB project as an alternative model for accomplishing social goals.

During the 1960s and 1970s, along with expanding the center's physical plant, I was active in the movement to restructure state government to aid the blind. Although we had abandoned the idea of a separate agency for the blind in

133

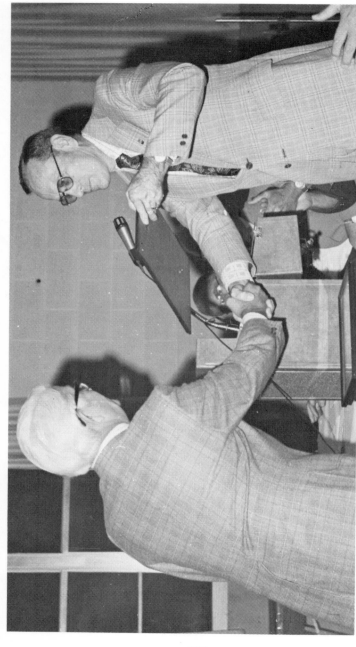

Outgoing AEB president (left) Lawson Glover of Malvern, congratulates Dr. James M. Fowler of Little Rock, the new president of AEB's board and the 67th president of Lions International.

the early fifties as a result of the controversy with the rehabilitation counselors, by the early 1960s it was apparent that blind people were still not getting their fair share of rehabilitation funds. Thus, in 1965 I suggested that instead of pushing for a separate agency or commission for the blind, we try to promote a bill establishing a separate division in the Education Department. Since the early conflict, Ashley Ross had died and had been succeeded as Director of Vocational Rehabilitation by Don Russell. Although thirty-four states already had separate divisions for the blind, Russell vehemently opposed all efforts to establish such a system in Arkansas.

I had hoped that by asking for a division rather than a separate agency, the education lobby would not contest the change. Russell, however, felt threatened by the proposed legislation and vowed to do everything possible to prevent passage of the bill. At one point he even spoke to the AEB board and accused me of being a disruptive influence in the work for the blind in the state.

Despite Russell's opposition, we proceeded with our plan. We conducted a survey which revealed that a majority of the members of the Arkansas legislature were Lions Club members. Under the direction of Byrl Byles we circulated our proposal, discussed it and recruited legislators to our cause. Finally the bill passed the legislature, received the governor's signature and became law and after twenty-six years, Arkansas had a separate division to serve the blind.

During the first year of operation under the new system, we doubled the number of blind people served, proving the point I had been trying to make for years — that under the general rehabilitation program, the blind had not been receiving their fair share of the rehabilitation dollar.

Sadly, in 1970, under Governor Dale Bumpers's governmental reorganization program, the separate division was abandoned and the programs for the blind were placed in the Department of Human Services. In 1975, though, we sponsored another bill creating the Office for the Blind and Visually Impaired, which again gave the blind people of the state an autonomous division, this time under the Commission for Rehabilitation. Under this system the newly created office for the blind could not be merged with other offices by executive order, but only by another act of the legislature.

I couldn't be more pleased with the new system. I had been the first and, for a while, the only full-time employee who worked to aid the adult blind in Arkansas. Now there were over 200 full time workers in the state employed by the various public and private agencies, offering the blind people of Arkansas a wide variety of needed services.

Along with these important changes in the structure of state government and the increase in workers for the blind, the 1960s and 1970s were decades of tremendous physical growth for our rehabilitation center. Through the generosity of individuals like Jess Odom, Robert Sakon, Grace Pinkerton and others along with the aid and cooperation of national and state agencies, we expanded from the Brack Home to a modern six-building complex guarded by our symbolic lion. But the changes in our facilities told only half of the history of the AEB's growth during that era. The other half of the story involved the changes in the programs that we conducted inside those wonderful buildings.

CHAPTER 9

Farewell to the Tin Cup

An ancient Hebrew proverb says if you give a hungry man a fish, he eats for a day, but if you teach him to be a fisherman, he will never be hungry again. The truth of that adage became evident to me during the early years of the center's operation. Even though my original concept of the facility had focused on prevocational adjustment, I soon realized we would have to expand our horizons to include vocational training as well.

Most trainees arrive at the AEB confused and uncertain as to how they will ever earn a living. To learn to travel independently and take care of personal needs are certainly essential, but the ability to be economically self-sufficient is a paramount concern. To meet this need, our trainees undergo a series of tests to determine their abilities and aptitudes and participate in a job observation program to introduce them to other blind people who are successfully engaged in a variety of occupations.

Traditionally, blind people worked in a few limited occupations such as vending stand operator, masseur, chiropractor, salesman or piano tuner. In the last two decades, however, a virtual revolution has occurred in work opportunities for the blind. With over 5,000 different jobs filled successfully by blind people, we constantly needed to expand and update our vocational training at the center as well as establish new programs to meet the unique needs of our trainees.

One of the AEB's most innovative vocational programs resulted from a casual invitation. At least once a month the center sponsored a banquet luncheon to help the trainees develop necessary dining skills and hear various individuals from the community deliver brief speeches following the meal. In 1966 I invited a friend who worked for the Internal Revenue

Service to attend our banquet and speak to the group on income tax problems. My friend asked if he could bring Fred Johnson, the state director of the IRS, because he said Johnson had expressed an interest in our program and wanted to see how our facility operated.

Following the luncheon, I escorted Mr. Johnson on a tour of the center. While we strolled around the grounds he told me about a close friend of his who had been an accountant and gone blind. His friend had encountered difficulties in finding a job and Mr. Johnson had become interested in the vocational training of the visually handicapped. Toward the end of our walk he told me about a new program initiated by the IRS where taxpayers could telephone from all over the state for information regarding their taxes. "You know, Roy," Mr. Johnson said, "a blind person could be trained to be a taxpayer service representative and help us with all these telephone calls."

Of course opening up an entire new vocational field for the blind was an exciting prospect. Soon after our talk, Mr. Johnson held a series of meetings in both Little Rock and Washington, D. C. to explore the possibilities of training and employing blind taxpayer service representatives. I attended almost all of the sessions as did Mr. Johnson; J. O. Murphy, the Director of Research and Training at the AEB; Douglas MacFarland, the Director of the Office for the Blind; George Magers, the assistant director; Nicholas W. Williams, the coordinator for the Employment of the Handicapped of the IRS; and L. H. Autry, the director of the state program for the blind. As a result of these conferences the Arkansas Enterprises for the Blind received a six-month grant from the federal rehabilitation service to establish a pilot program to teach blind persons to become taxpayer assistants.

Our first concern was to find some bright, qualified blind persons for the first Taxpayer Service Representative (TSR) class. Unfortunately, several rehabilitation counselors in Arkansas misunderstood the purpose of the new project and referred individuals whom they had been unable to place in any other employment. I explained to the counselors that we needed blind individuals with high IQs, excellent memories and vocabulary as well as the desire and the ability to improve their mobility, independent living and communication skills.

I actually had one particular candidate in mind. I felt Jack McSpadden would be a perfect pioneer to open this new avenue of employment for the blind. A native of Batesville, Jack lost the sight of his left eye after being struck with a baseball when he was in the fourth grade. Three years later he lost his right eye when a fence post rolled off a truck and hit him in the face. He had finished the school for the blind and earned a college degree before completing our vocational evaluation program at the center. Unable to find employment, he was referred by his rehabilitation counselor to our vocational evaluation program at the center. Toward the end of the evaluation process, I approached him about the new TSR program.

Jack accepted the challenge and started the training program with two other individuals. One person dropped out early and only Jack and a young lady completed the course. Fred Johnson quickly offered both graduates a temporary appointment with the local IRS office but after six months of handling as many as 100 phone calls a day only Jack qualified for permanent appointment with the Internal Revenue Service.

The Department of Health, Education and Welfare extended our grant for an additional three years and we refined our course of study to include automatic data processing and role playing sessions to augment the basic income tax information material. After fourteen years, the program had become one of our strongest vocational training projects. Through the cooperation of the AEB, the Internal Revenue Service, the state Office for the Blind and Visually Impaired and the federal government, 230 blind persons have graduated from the program and found employment in fifty-nine different IRS offices.

Leonard Robinson, in his autobiography *Light at the Tunnel End*, used a quotation from IRS Commissioner Johnnie M. Walters that reflected not only the success of our TSR classes but also the extent to which the program became mutually beneficial to both blind people and the IRS. "The success of our blind Taxpayer Service Representatives is indeed a study in courage and achievement" Walters said. "It is a fulfillment of a sort of American dream and proof that the Revenue Service does have a soul."

As Americans enter the 1980s, a single technological instrument is revolutionizing the way we live, the way we work, the way we travel and even the way we organize our leisure time. Only a brief quarter of a century ago, computers were regarded as the futuristic pipe dream of a handful of engineers and science fiction writers. Today, however, not only are computers considered a necessity by businesses of all sizes and complexities, but the era of computers for home use appears to be close at hand.

This revolution has generated a series of exciting occupational opportunities for blind people. As early as 1963, the industry designed computers to produce printouts in braille and since that time, an increasing number of blind individuals have been trained to operate sophisticated computer equipment.

Recognizing the enormous potential for the blind in the field of computer programming, I began investigating the possibility of making computer training part of our vocational program in 1973 and by the end of the decade, the AEB offered one of the largest and most comprehensive programs in the country to teach blind and visually impaired individuals to be computer programmers.

Our program continues to utilize the most up-to-date equipment including a Honeywell 6/36 computer which provides training in COBOL, RPG and FORTRAN languages, an LED-120, and several video terminals with screens, closed circuit viewers and a voice synthesizer.

Despite rising unemployment, every individual who has completed our computer course has found a job. Recently, we were particularly proud of Becky Henry who, after finishing our program, became the first totally blind computer programmer employed at Disney World in Florida. Everyone connected with the AEB has great hope that Becky's success will help pave the way for future graduates of our computer training course to find jobs with private industry as well as with the government agencies. As soon as possible, the AEB plans to expand its offerings in this area to enable even more blind people to be in the center of the computer revolution.

Since financing innovative vocational education programs has presented a serious obstacle to the employment of the blind, over the years I maintained several contacts with our friends in the federal government who were involved with appropriations for rehabilitation research and training. In 1973, through the combined efforts of myself and United States Senator John McClellan of Arkansas, the AEB received a grant from the Rehabilitation Services Administration of HEW to train Civil Service Information Specialists for the U.S. Civil Service Commission. A few years later, we expanded the project to fill a variety of information expediter jobs in private industry.

The early results of this "Project with Industry" included identifying several jobs for blind people with the South-western Bell Telephone Company and a program demonstrating the feasibility of training blind information service specialists to access computer stored data through synthetic speech. We placed many of our graduates from the program in the thirty-eight regional offices of the General Services Administration. The United States government established these offices to provide information to business and government agencies as well as the general public. Our graduates, who were well versed in the complexities of governmental services, referred the various callers to the proper federal, state or local government agencies capable of supplying assistance.

Because of the success of the "Project with Industry," in 1978 the AEB launched a Community Service Advisor program to produce qualified workers to fill the rapidly growing need for ombudsmen — knowledgeable individuals who listen to the public's complaints about bureaucratic dilemmas and offer advice or, if necessary, refer them to the proper government or private agency. Our intensive community advisor course trained qualified blind persons in regulations for consumer protection, landlord-tenant relations, requirements for Social Security benefits, Medicare, Medicaid and food stamps.

While not all of the AEB vocational programs operate on such a large scale, each one is designed to expand the economic horizons of the blind people referred to the center by the rehabilitation agency. We want to impress upon our trainess that they are no longer occupationally restricted to the traditional "blind trades." One example of this expansion of vocational education was our Small Business Management training course that began in 1974. The course teaches blind persons the basics of good business practices such as inventory control, salesmanship, stocking and stock rotation, banking, insurance, tax codes and bookkeeping. By 1980 fifty-one graduates of the program had launched their careers. Although most of them work for the state-operated business enterprise program, a few have gone into business for themselves.

Later we inaugurated a small engine repair course to teach blind people with the necessary manual dexterity to repair lawn mowers, tillers, outboard motors, chain saws and other small machines. Combining this program with our small business training course, we enabled our trainees to establish their own small engine repair shops.

I see enormous potential for blind and visually impaired people in the area of small motor repair and maintenance and hope our program proves as successful as one of our oldest vocational programs — training switchboard operators and receptionists. Visitors to any office, whether a private business or a state agency, receive their first impression from the receptionist. Telephone callers also receive their initial perception of a company from their experience with the switchboard operator. I always felt that blind people could compete with their sighted counterparts in this type of work and consequently in 1960 we instituted a training program in this area.

By 1977 this project had led us to the threshhold of a breakthrough in opportunities for the blind. That spring, Ann McDaniel, a twenty-one-year-old graduate of the AEB's switchboard program, began training with the Bell Telephone Company for a job as a long-distance operator.

Up until that time, a blind person had never been a long distance operator anywhere in the country. In order to alter this situation, Ann used a special computer manufactured at the Massachusetts Institute of Technology in cooperation with the telephone company and the AEB. The machine cost over $50,000, which was paid for by a grant from the "Project with Industry." I believed that the money on the experimental computer would be well invested if Ann succeeded and thereby opened the door to jobs never before available to the blind.

A long-distance console consisted of eighty-two buttons arranged in eight rows. When a sighted operator received a call, red, yellow or white lights flashed across the board, signaling the information the operator needed to successfully complete the call. The computer was plugged into the console and the machine converted the information into a thin strip of pins that tickled Ann's fingers, telling her in braille what she needed to know — if the caller had dialed 0, or wanted to call station-to-station or person-to-person, or wanted to call collect or use a credit card.

I had great confidence in Ann's ability to become a long distance operator. Blind since birth, she had attended the state school for the blind in Louisiana but had transferred to public school where she had demonstrated her academic ability. She came to the AEB in 1974 and upon completion of her training, accepted a position as a switchboard operator at Southwestern Bell in Little Rock.

On June 7, 1977 my faith in Ann McDaniel was rewarded when she became the first blind long-distance operator in the Bell System. That day generated considerable excitement at both the phone company and the AEB. I had worked closely with the Rehabilitation Services Administration and their statisticians estimated that between 200 and 300 blind people could work as telephone operators throughout the United States if they had access to the experimental computer Ann used.

I also realized the new computer could open up avenues for blind people in related areas in which information needed to be transmitted or retrieved by computer. These opportunities seemed light years away from the traditional blind trades. Ann McDaniel's success multiplied the chances for other blind people to become an active part of the technological revolution and I wanted the AEB to remain in the forefront of developing these new advances.

In the next few years we expanded our programs to develop technologically based clerical skills. For example, we started a medical transcriptionist course that included the study of medical terminology, anatomy and physiology, and the organization and preparation of medical reports. Word processing also became an important part of our curricula. Our instructors have access to a wide variety of up-to-date machines such as an IBM System Six and an IBM Audio Typing Unit to keep our trainees competitive in the open job market.

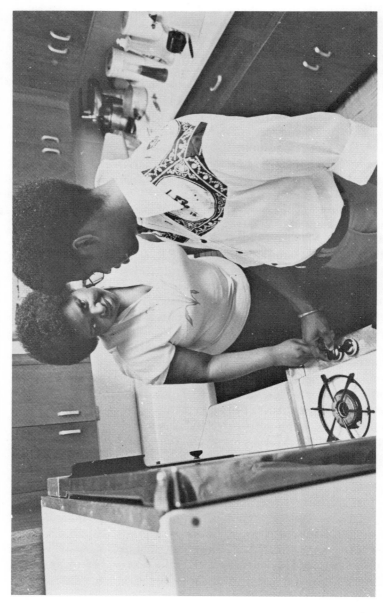

A trainee at AEB receives instruction in cooking skills in the course Techniques of Daily Living.

Through progress in technology, generous government funding and our own initiative, we have tried to make the AEB in Little Rock one of the best vocational education facilities for the adult blind in the country. Recognizing the enormous potential of technology in opening new occupational opportunities for the blind, we have tried to be a leader in creating innovative training programs. Our ultimate goal is to relegate the image of the blind beggar to a long-ago past, say farewell to his tin cup and produce a group of highly skilled blind employees who will assume responsible positions in both government and private industry.

Over the past three decades, vocational training has been only one area in which we have expanded the services offered by the center. From the time of my youth in Ironton, I recognized the necessity of change. Institutions that refuse to change wither away. Thus, we have continuously added new programs to our core of orientation and mobility, daily living techniques, communications skills and social and recreational activities. For example, in 1962 we opened an optical aids clinic to help people with low vision utilize their limited sight. A $6,000 grant from the Office of Vocational Rehabilitation and the Arkansas Rehabilitation Service furnished our initial equipment and for almost twenty years the clinic has provided eye examinations and dispensed low vision aids such as magnifiers and bifocals to over 300 people annually.

In order to aid the largest number of blind people possible, over the years the AEB added a series of training courses and institutes for rehabilitation counselors and home teachers. I have long been an advocate of professional training for workers in the field and have supported stronger accreditation standards, intern programs and beneficial in-service training. To this end, the AEB has developed a symbiotic relationship with the University of Arkansas at Little Rock.

Originally my alma mater — Little Rock Junior College — UALR has blossomed into a fine urban university with almost 10,000 students. I worked closely with university officials for over thirteen years and in 1977 UALR announced the inauguration of a master's degree program to train professional workers for the blind. We established the program with a grant from the Rehabilitation Services Administration that was secured under the auspices of the AEB. The center also

145

aided the new program by offering a series of internships to train orientation and mobility instructors and rehabilitation teachers to help the students become familiar with rehabilitation of the blind.

The movement for professional education in the field of mobility instruction actually evolved rather slowly. The first graduate program in mobility did not appear until 1960 when Boston College offered the first degree plan. A year later Western Michigan University launched a similar program and for several years these were the only two institutions that provided formal training for mobility instructors.

While overall I certainly favor educational programs like the ones offered at Boston College, Western Michigan, UALR and other schools, there are some inherent dangers in over-specializing orientation and mobility instructors. One of these problems became clear to me after the national accreditation organization, over my objection, stipulated that a person must have 20/20 vision in order to be a mobility instructor. What that qualification meant was that under this new system, Oliver Burke, who had taught mobility to more blind people than anyone in the country, would not have been eligible for the new university graduate programs.

My objection is not to professionalism in general but rather to narrow and sometimes pompous specialization. Even the new terminology in the field seems designed to make what we do sound excessively complicated. The professionals rejected terms like "mobility technician" or "mobility specialist" and instead adopted the name "peripathologist," a derivative of "peripathology" which literally means "the science of walking around." Such barriers of standards and jargon do little to improve our basic goal of serving the blind.

At the AEB I have always followed the philosophy that we are a "trainee-centered" institution — our only purpose is to serve blind clients. I always shudder when I come in contact with "staff-oriented" programs where scheduling and other decisions are reached with the convenience of professional staff as the highest priority.

My reservations concerning professionalism in the field are matched by my concern in another area that affects the work for the blind — mainstreaming or placing blind children in a regular school situation. I have many friends on both sides of this issue and recognize the validity of each of their arguments. My friends who favor separate residential schools argue that blind children in public schools are never really accepted by their sighted classmates and that public school teachers lack the training to work with blind children and tend to either spend too much or too little time with them.

On the other hand, a strong case can be made that by attending a separate residential school a blind child is deprived of the daily affection of his or her family and suffers isolation from the sighted world, which is tantamount to being divorced from reality.

Frankly, I used to be a strong advocate of mainstreaming. Over the last few years, however, I have had some second thoughts on the matter. With the passage of recent laws (P.L. 94142) and mainstreaming handicapped children into regular classroom situations, I have begun to wonder if perhaps expectations are being raised too high. Most public schools lack proper equipment and specially trained teachers to meet the needs of blind children. Most teachers still have a tendency to regard any minor academic accomplishment by a blind child as a major educational breakthrough, and sighted classmates still regard blind children as "different," making little effort to include them in school activities. More and more, however, the parents of blind children expect the public schools to take complete charge of the training and preparation of their child to function in a sighted world. The public schools are simply not equipped to accomplish this task. While I recognize that there are no "right" answers for every blind child, I do believe we need to approach the mainstreaming of blind young people with a healthy skepticism. Also, with the improvement of residential schools in terms of facilities, staff and instruction, the parents of blind children now have more of a choice as to which type of school will best meet the educational needs of their child.

While issues like mainstreaming and professional education are a source of endless debate among my colleagues in the field, medical advances designed to restore sight are universally applauded. Some of my happiest moments in my forty years of working for the blind have concerned my involvement in efforts to facilitate sight restoration.

147

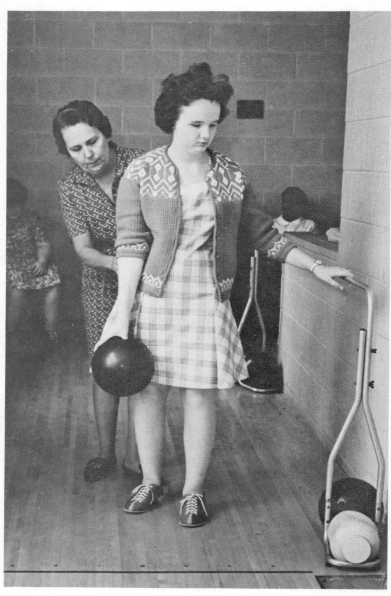

Among AEB's many recreational activities is bowling using a one-lane alley donated by the Pine Bluff Evening Lions Club in 1964.

On a chilling pre-dawn morning in January, 1979 a transportation network swung into action from its base in Little Rock. Under a police escort two men in an ambulance whisked a small styrofoam box through the fog to the airport across town. The men transferred the box to an airline pilot who kept the container by his side in the cockpit of the plane until he reached his destination in New Orleans where another ambulance picked up the tiny cargo.

The box contained a pair of human eyes for two recipients of cornea transplants. The tightly coordinated transportation system was necessary because eyes must be enucleated (removed) within six hours after the death of a donor and must be transplanted within twenty-four hours. The cornea is the transplant tissue which covers the iris and only one cornea transplant (whole eyeballs are not transplanted) is allowed a recipient at any one time because eyes are extremely scarce.

Later that January day, an eighty-five-year-old woman who had been blind since her twenties received one of the corneas and eventually saw three generations of her offspring for the first time. The second cornea saved the sight of a four-year-old girl who had been blinded in an automobile accident. Both corneas were provided by the Arkansas Eye and Kidney Bank, a sight conservation project of the state's Lions Clubs.

Like my connection with the AEB, I became involved in the early inception of the Eye Bank. I had always been as concerned with the prevention of blindness as about the rehabilitation of the permanently blind because I knew that, had there been a decent sight conservation program when I first experienced trouble with my own eyes, I would never have been blind. Obviously, the best rehabilitation is the restoration of sight.

Although cornea transplants had been available in other areas for some time, Arkansas had never had a transplant program until Dr. Fritz Fraunfelder became the chairman of the Ophthalmology Department at the University of Arkansas Medical Center in Little Rock. The medical facility also employed a young doctor named Pat Flannigan who had been having some success with kidney transplants. In the early 1970s the two doctors influenced Harlan Lane, a local banker, to raise enough money to create the Tissue and Organ Foundation of Arkansas.

149

Because of my work at the AEB, Lane invited me to serve on the board of the new foundation. At one of our early meetings a member of the board indicated he had visited several eye banks in other states and they all seemed to be sponsored by the local Lions Clubs. Several of our members then suggested the Arkansas Lions Clubs might be a logical sponsor for the Eye Bank in our state.

I approached the Lions State Committee for Sight Conservation with the proposal and after considerable debate the committee recommended that the Lions adopt the Eye Bank as a statewide project in coordination with the medical center. A few months later the Lions state convention adopted the idea and the Eye and Kidney Bank became the Arkansas Lions' second statewide project.

The Lions' role in the Eye Bank has been to publicize its activities and influence the public to will eyes and kidneys to the foundation. The Lions have also promoted legislation to create an easier method for an individual to will parts of his body to be used for medical purposes after the donor's death. This legislation includes a place on all Arkansas driver's licenses where a person can indicate his wishes in this regard and a donor card, which in case of an automobile or other accident, can be used to insure that eyes or kidneys will be left to the Eye and Kidney Bank.

One of the advantages the foundation has brought to Arkansas has been participation in a nationwide Eye Bank Network. If an eye is donated in Little Rock and we do not have an immediate applicant, but a doctor in Kansas City or Baltimore or New Orleans is requesting one, the eye can be shipped immediately to aid a needy recipient.

For several years the foundation's board always met at the AEB and at one point several members recommended me as the new president of the board. I suggested we should nominate one of our lay leaders and as a result Herman West, a member of the Lions International board, became president while I agreed to assume the position of treasurer of the tissue foundation board.

At first our staff at the center kept the records for the EKB and aided in the administration of the program. Eventually the Lions began raising around $40,000 annually to support the project. The expense of the program caused several people

150

to ask me if I thought the Lions could afford two statewide endeavors. I strongly believed they could and regarded both the Eye Bank and the rehabilitation center as important components in the state's efforts to aid the blind.

A few years ago I withdrew from active participation in the Eye Bank program to allow more people to become involved in the Lions work for the blind. In my opinion, between the EKB and the AEB, the Lions of Arkansas have devoted themselves to a consistent theme of helping the visually handicapped and have earned the title of "Knights of the Blind."

As late as 1966, *Reader's Digest* carried an advertisement by the Better Vision Institute showing a blind man walking down a street with a white cane in one hand and a tin cup in the other hand. A sign on his back read "My Days are Darker Than Your Nights." Like most of my colleagues in the field, I found the ad offensive and appalling because of its message that blind people cannot be independent and are forever lost in a world of darkness.

Regrettably, not every blind person can have his sight restored by a cornea transplant, but nevertheless, I hope with the passage of time that new advertisements will appear showing blind people hard at work as taxpayer service representatives or computer programmers or long distance telephone operators or small business managers. These ads will convey a new message — that blind people are skilled and productive citizens and not a class of street beggars. This is an important message that is needed to destroy a cruel stereotype and allow blind people to say once and for all, farewell to the tin cup.

CHAPTER 10
Before the 21st Century

Any person deprived of sight in the 1980s has an excellent opportunity to enjoy a happy and meaningful existence. No longer are blind people relegated to a few limited vocational choices or denied access to educational and recreational materials to enhance the quality of their lives. Two highly significant factors that have made this improved situation possible are first, the movement for standards and accreditation among institutions that aid the blind and second, the numerous new technologies that have expanded blind people's ability to function in the everyday world.

Not too long ago, unthinking and sometimes unscrupulous individuals engaged in tear-jerk, sob-story fundraising campaigns to aid the blind. Many times the only people who received any "help" were the fundraisers themselves. These scam artists roamed freely through various charities exploiting both the handicapped and the public at large. But slowly this circumstance changed. Reform-minded individuals began to demand a system of standards: a system of accreditation that would assure blind people quality training and treatment at the various agencies throughout the country.

My first encounter with some rather shady dealings in the field involved an organization called the Arkansas Lighthouse for the Blind. The public usually regards the term "lighthouse" as an excellent name for an agency serving the visually handicapped. Workers in the movement, however, often disagree. The use of the word goes back many years to two sisters, wealthy New York socialites, who in their travels encountered some blind persons in Europe making and selling small craft objects. Returning home, these matrons started a comparable project in which they taught blind beggars to weave baskets and carpets which the blind people could sell on the streets.

Since the operation accorded far more dignity than begging, the ladies embraced the idea that their philanthropy offered a "lighthouse" to the unfortunates in the dark.

A lighthouse is a signal that danger is near and that is precisely what it came to mean among those involved in helping the blind. "Lighthouse" caught on with the public and newer programs began using the designation for its fundraising potential. Unfortunately, many of these programs degenerated into fronts for unethical solicitations and over the years "lighthouse" became a disreputable term, even though today there are some accredited agencies for the blind that still utilize the designation.

In Arkansas, a charismatic blind preacher named Jeff Smith promoted the first lighthouse. I met the Reverend Jeff at a chapel service during my student days at the School for the Blind. He was an old-fashioned spellbinder, an ambitious and educated individual who had attended Southern Methodist University. Reverend Jeff impressed me so much that some years later I invited him to speak to our alumni association. At that meeting he conducted an inspirational evening and even added a musical touch by singing and playing the saw.

Around this time I was opening the first vending stands and while I had great hopes for the program, I knew it could not meet the vocational needs of all the blind people in the state. Consequently, I had another idea. I wanted to open a workshop to manufacture brooms and mops in the old school for the blind building at Eighteenth and Center. The school had moved to its new location on Markham and I felt the workshop would be an excellent use of the facility. At our alumni meeting I discovered Reverend Jeff had an interest in a similar project. Earlier in his career he had actually founded a workshop in Fort Worth, Texas, and I had high hopes he would be helpful in getting our project off the ground.

A few months later I tried unsuccessfully for a legislative appropriation for the workshop and when that failed I became discouraged about the possibility of acquiring adequate financial support. Almost immediately Reverend Jeff phoned and said he could raise the money through private sources and I, rather naively, transferred all my files to him. Reverend Jeff then created a board of directors and began soliciting money for his proposed lighthouse.

153

I assumed the project was proceeding as planned until one day a friend of mine who was a field consultant for the American Foundation for the Blind came by my office. After a little hemming and hawing she finally asked, "Roy, have you ever checked any of Jeff Smith's references?"

"Why no," I replied. "He's a preacher and attended college and . . ."

"If you were investing your own money, wouldn't you check?"

"Well, sure . . ." I did check. I wrote to the Junior League of Fort Worth, the sponsoring organization of Reverend Jeff's Lighthouse in Texas. I received an immediate reply informing me that under no circumstances could the organization recommend Jeff Smith. While he had been associated with them, he had kept virtually no records or ledgers and upon his dismissal he had been unable to account for over $10,000.

By this time Reverend Jeff had interested Governor Homer Adkins in the workshop and when I showed the letter from Texas to Welfare Commissioner John Pipkin, he asked me not to reveal the information to the governor. Governor Adkins had embraced the idea and wanted to give Smith a $5,000 revolving fund utilizing the state building grounds. At that moment I feared that the blind were not going to receive the help they deserved and the work for the blind was about to get buried in an avalanche of bad publicity.

Therefore, I went to see Reverend Jeff and told him I knew about the debacle in Texas. I also said I realized anyone could make an honest mistake, but now he had an opportunity to make an important contribution to the work for the visually handicapped in Arkansas and I assured him I would be willing to help in any way I could.

Reverend Jeff never asked for my help. The vending stand program took more and more of my time and my other commitments gradually forced me to let him run the workshop his own way. The whole thing broke my heart. Reverend Jeff was a cynic who believed in the old idea of telling people all kinds of sob stories to raise money. Once I ran across him in downtown Little Rock and he told me, "Roy, you know I've tried preaching; I've tried evangelism; and I've tried some other things, but nothing, and I mean nothing, gets into the pockets of rich folks like helping the blind."

154

On the surface, the Lighthouse appeared successful. But underneath, the operation was not what it appeared to be. Even though Reverend Jeff raised a tremendous amount of money, the blind people who worked in the shop received few benefits. Instead, Reverend Jeff forced them to work long hours for little pay and the Lighthouse became a philanthropic scam. Unfortunately, the very success of Smith's unethical fundraising made it difficult for me to publicly critize him. If I challenged the preacher, my comments would look like the whining of a jealous rival.

At the beginning of World War II, much to my chagrin, the Reverend expanded his operation. Although the war limited access to many raw materials, Reverend Jeff managed to get a defense contract to make brooms, which entitled him to special certificates for corn. One reliable source alleged that the Lighthouse shipped car loads of substandard brooms to places like the Brooklyn Navy Yard, where the brooms were rejected because they failed to meet government specifications. Reverend Jeff then hopped a train for New York and sold the brooms on the civilian market at outrageously high prices. Despite a later investigation, the money obtained from these sales never appeared in the records of the Arkansas Lighthouse.

While today the Lighthouse in Arkansas is a reputable operation, furnishing many employment opportunities for the blind, my experience with Reverend Jeff taught me the importance of having standards or accreditation among the agencies involved with the visually handicapped. I think the Lighthouse was also one of the reasons I turned to the Lions Clubs for the rehabilitation center's board of directors. I knew these men would be active and responsible and would account to the public. I wanted accountability in our operation because people are too often cheated by seemingly good causes. Even to this day the image of the Lighthouse remains the symbol of an honest charity and over the years I know many people have contributed money to the Lighthouse thinking they made a donation to our program.

Unfortunately, the charities for the blind have always drawn a share of scam artists and con men. Another example I always remember was an individual who set up a foundation to train dog guides and raised over $60,000 in donations before an alert state legislator discovered he did not have a single dog or trainer. Because this type of scandal was not uncommon in the work for the blind, many concerned professionals, including myself, set out in the early 1950s to establish some safeguards to discourage a new generation of exploiters.

The creation of uniform standards among the agencies for the blind, however, was not an easy task. Unlike other charities such as the American Heart Association or the American Cancer Society, the efforts to aid the visually handicapped have never generated a single nationwide organization to oversee its activities. Instead, the work for the blind has been characterized by an ever-increasing and often competitive group of organizations. One directory currently lists over 400 separate associations working for the blind in various capacities. Probably the most celebrated organization is the American Foundation for the Blind. Founded in 1921, the AFB disseminates information about the nature of blindness, conducts workshops and seminars and acts as the most powerful lobbying group on behalf of people without sight. But the AFB has never had the resources to ultimately coordinate all of the various organizations, and when the efforts for standards and accreditation began, the Foundation would not achieve this goal on its own initiative.

The first decisive thrust for the establishment of standards came during my term as president of the American Association of Workers for the Blind in 1951. At the convention in Daytona Beach, Florida, we adopted a resolution to appoint a committee to study the creation of a seal of good practice or code of ethics, especially in the area of fundraising. The following year at our Louisville, Kentucky convention the committee submitted a favorable report but the idea encountered considerable opposition. Representatives of several small agencies saw the specter of someone monitoring and criticizing their operations as a potential threat and managed to delay any action on the matter.

In 1953 I chaired a lengthy and tumultuous meeting at the AAWB convention in Washington, D.C. Although the opposition remained strong, we outvoted the smaller groups and created a board to award a seal of good practice to agencies that maintained certain standards in fundraising, public relations and educational programs. While I was not naive enough to believe the seal concept would solve all our problems, I did feel optimistic that we had taken a giant step in the right direction.

The idea of accountability to the public gained momentum in the late 1950s and early 1960s. In 1956 at a seminar in New Orleans sponsored by the American Foundation for the Blind and the Office of Vocational Rehabilitation, we established guidelines to govern the growth of rehabilitation centers. Then in 1963 the AFB, in conjunction with other organizations, created a commission to formulate standards and create an independent accreditation agency. Financed by a variety of foundations, the Commission on Standards and Accreditation of Services for the Blind (COMSTAC) began its work in February, 1964. I received an invitation to serve on the COMSTAC committee dealing with rehabilitation centers and I gratefully accepted what I regarded as an opportunity to become a part of one of the most significant events in the history of the blind. Agencies aiding the visually handicapped had existed in the United States for over 150 years and yet there had been no basic standard for the delivery of services. As a result, the flimflammers had always been able to exploit the situation. But with COMSTAC we planned to do something to stop them.

In January, 1967 our dream became a reality. Based on the final report issued by COMSTAC, the National Accreditation Council for Agencies Serving the Blind and Visually Handicapped began operation that month. NAC, as the organization is more commonly known, received its initial funding from the American Foundation for the Blind and the Department of Health, Education and Welfare. Eventually the council hoped to become independent through funds raised from accredited institutions and endowments. NAC acts as the accrediting agency for institutions that provide direct services to blind people — rehabilitation centers, workshops, residential schools and training centers for dog guides.

Accreditation by NAC signified that an agency had met nationally accepted standards of quality services in the areas of training, management and ethical fundraising. To receive NAC accreditation, an institution had to undergo a period of self-study followed by a rigorous examination by a visiting team of experts. In the first ten years of existence NAC extended this accreditation to over sixty agencies across the United States.

As the director of the Arkansas Enterprises for the Blind, I wanted our institution to seek accreditation and demonstrate that we had no fear of anyone visiting our facility and scrutinizing our program. The AEB had annually received the "Seal of Good Practice" from the American Association of Workers for the Blind since 1957 and seeing in NAC an opportunity to expand our reputation for quality services, I filed the necessary accreditation paper soon after the national association's founding.

In February, 1970, at a board meeting at the Marion Hotel, I proudly announced that the Arkansas Enterprises for the Blind had become the first rehabilitation center in the nation to earn accreditation from NAC. In making the announcement I told the board, "Now the rehabilitation counselors who refer their clients to our agency are assured that they will receive the best training available." I had never felt more satisfaction in all my years with the AEB.

The process that culminated in our accreditation was a demanding one. At the conclusion of a year-long self-study that involved many board members as well as our staff, a six-man team of specialists from NAC spent three days at the AEB conducting their own investigation. Once at the center, the NAC team interviewed every employee, checked our personnel records, reviewed our bookkeeping and thoroughly inspected the physical plant. The NAC representatives were exhaustive in their efforts, and agencies which received their approval could confidently say they offered the highest quality services available.

Since I had long been an advocate of strict standards, I gladly served two terms on the board of directors of the National Accreditation Council. I chaired several on-site evaluation teams, an experience I always found rewarding because of the personal involvement in assisting other agencies to improve the delivery of quality services to the blind. For too many years people like Reverend Jeff Smith exploited both blind people and the general public because of a lack of accreditation agencies. Thus, the establishment of NAC proved to be a momentous step forward in policing the organizations serving the blind.

While accreditation resulted in vastly improved services, the development of technological aids has had a revolutionary impact on the lives of blind people over the last few decades. By utilizing these devices, the blind have been able to gain employment in areas that have traditionally been closed to them and discover numerous recreational outlets to enrich the quality of their lives. Rather than fearing technology as some social critics advocate, the blind welcome new and improved machines as the servants of mankind and view the future with hopeful anticipation. I personally share this optimism, primarily because of the miraculous technological advances I have witnessed throughout my own lifetime. When I first suffered the ravages of trachoma in 1918, not even radio existed to help a blind person combat the lonely hours. Now the possibilities seem almost unlimited.

One of the earliest advances in technological aids for the blind — and one that I still use extensively — was the talking book, either a phonograph or a magnetic tape player. Developed by the Research Department of the American Foundation for the Blind, talking books opened the world of reading and hence the world of ideas and knowledge to millions of blind people who lacked the skills to read braille. Over the last fifty years, not only have the machines themselves been refined but the availability of material has dramatically increased. A legally blind person, upon application to the local library for the blind, is automatically eligible to receive a talking book machine and the Library of Congress, which designates state library commissions or other public libraries as lending agencies for the blind, supplies a lengthy list of titles available on long-playing records and tapes. Our own library at the Arkansas Enterprises for the Blind contains hundreds of recorded works ranging from established classics of English literature to western novels, science fiction thrillers and current magazines. These recordings give our trainees access to a miscellany of new experiences that years ago would have been beyond the reach of visually handicapped individuals.

When we first opened the rehabilitation center in 1947, our technological aids consisted of the typewriter and the brailler. The brailler represented an improvement over the slate and stylus (a device that enabled the writer to punch out one braille dot at a time) because it could produce an entire letter at once. The brailler was to writing braille what a typewriter is to longhand. At first, we relied on a brailler called the Perkins Writer which was developed by the research division of the Perkins School for the Blind. A few years later we acquired a Thermoform machine — a device that made duplicate copies of braille material. The staff considered this device a tremendous innovation because we could produce multiple copies of educational material on the premises of the center.

By the early 1950s federal money for research increased and more and more effort went into developing an electronic machine that could read print for the blind. This attempt produced the sterotoner — a machine based on the idea that printed characters could make individualized beeping sounds. I never believed the stereotoner would be of much practical value and by and large I was right. But the machine was important because it led to something else and that something became one of the most important technological aids for the blind in the last twenty years.

Throughout my career in rehabilitation I have encountered many inventions to aid the visually handicapped. Some of these devices proved useful, others were impractical, and some were downright ridiculous. But of all the innovations I heard about over the years, none of them excited me as much as the Optacon. For the first time I saw the possibility of giving blind people direct access to printed matter — books, magazines, letters — without having to wait for someone else to transcribe the material into braille, record it or read it aloud.

The new machine utilized a miniature transistorized camera to scan the print and then reproduce an image of the actual letters using one hundred forty-four vibrating reeds or fibers which could be "read" with the fingertip. The term Optacon then was a contraction of optical and connection with tactile sense. John Linvill, a Stanford University engineering professor, who wanted to help his own blind daughter have quick access to printed school material, invented the device. Linvill teamed up with another Stanford researcher, James C. Bliss, to produce a refined model of the Optacon.

Developed by the Stanford Research Center, the machine was manufactured and marketed by Telesensory, Inc. Immediately after seeing a demonstration of the project, I called the people connected with the Optacon in California and in May,

1973, Telesensory designated the Arkansas Enterprises for the Blind as a training agency to instruct blind persons in the use of the Optacon. Although our staff did find the machine had some problems — for example, a congenitally blind person had no exposure to printed letters and a recently blinded individual often lacked the necessary sensitive touch — we also saw the tremendous potential of the device.

The first Optacon could only "read" print, not handwriting. Nevertheless, I saw in the machine the potential of allowing blind people to read their own mail, which had been a problem at the center from the beginning. While we stressed the dignity of independence to the trainees, the fact that someone else always had to read their personal correspondence aloud constantly undercut this notion. When we first opened the AEB, thoughtless staff members had occasionally read some rather intimate letters from families or lovers to trainees in the presence of other people. I stopped that practice and told our instructors that if anyone asked them to help with a letter to immediately find a private place to read the person's mail. But with the Optacon even that procedure would be unnecessary and the blind individual would receive an additional measure of independence.

While reading private correspondence is certainly important, the vocational opportunities inspired by the Optacon are staggering. The ability to immediately read office memos, letters and other job-related printed material could provide blind people access to hundreds of job opportunities that earlier had been closed to them.

In the area of technological advancement one innovation often leads to another and no sooner did we begin working with the Optacon than I heard about the possibility of a machine that could transcribe printed matter into the spoken word. At first, I thought a device to verbalize print came from the world of Flash Gordon or Buck Rogers, but in 1977 the AEB, because of its national reputation in the rehabilitation of the blind, was chosen as a testing location for the Kurzweil Reading Machine.

Marketed by the Boston-based Kurzweil Computer Company, the machine converts print into spoken English at the rate of 150 words per minute. An electronic control unit containing a digital tape operates the system and runs the scanner, which is essentially a camera that scans every letter

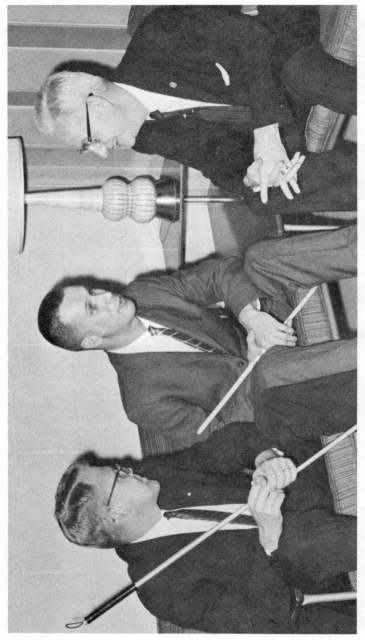

Dick Peters of Chicago (center), author of a column — "The Blind and You" — that appeared in the Lions magazine in the mid-60's, visited AEB in 1964. At left is A. B. "Bunk" Goodrum.

and punctuation mark. The scanner transmits images to a minicomputer which dissects the letters and groups them into words and then produces the speech sounds associated with each phonetic or basic unit of sound. The resulting synthesized speech closely resembles the monotonal speech of a deaf person.

The Kurzweil Reading Machine has all of the potential uses of the Optacon with the additional advantage of increased speed. To offset obsolescence, the manufacturers of the Optacon have recently produced a "Talking Optacon," although for the time being the high per unit cost limits the use of both talking machines to schools or other institutions. I am optimistic, however, that in the near future, technological advances will significantly reduce the cost, enabling more and more blind people to have immediate access to printed material.

At the AEB we already have some related instruments that have broadened the vocational opportunities for many of our trainees. For example, a closed circuit television scanner can enlarge print for those with limited vision. Private industry, through IBM, has contributed a "Talking Typewriter," which consists of a word processing system with an audio unit. This device permits blind secretaries to operate a word processing machine at a rate of speed equal to a sighted person.

Another important piece of equipment is the Speech Plus or Talking Calculator. Operating like a regular calculator, the instrument supplies the user with a verbal response. This device has been an invaluable tool for blind people going through the taxpayer representative program, the college preparatory course and other areas where mathematical calculation is important.

Making printed material readily available to the visually handicapped has also been the focus of one of my own recent projects. Since my retirement in 1978, I have devoted considerable energy to creating a Radio Reading Service for the Blind in Arkansas. Recognizing that expense places the Optacon and Kurzweil Reading Machine beyond the reach of the great majority of blind people, I believe that the radio can offer these individuals access to a sorely missed source of information — the daily newspaper.

Most blind people must depend on regular radio programs or television for local and national news. Unfortunately, most of this news, especially television news, tends to be superficial. Blind people also miss things like editorials, sports, marriage announcements, obituaries and other items of local interest that sighted people acquire through newspapers. To alleviate this situation the Radio Reading Service presents an individual reading the daily paper cover to cover on a special radio system. The blind person uses a closed circuit receiver in his home that is tuned to a special frequency. The broadcasts are provided by a subcarrier of a local FM station.

This service dates back to the 1960s when Stanley Potter, a blind ham radio operator who was also the Director of the Minnesota Service for the Blind, received a grant to establish a pilot program that included not only newspaper but magazine articles and even best-selling books. After hearing about the idea at an American Association of Workers for the Blind conference, I decided to call a meeting in Arkansas of representatives of various organizations in the rehabilitation field to see if we could pool our resources and establish a similar service.

Moved by an initial enthusiasm for the project, we elected a chairman to pursue the matter but a year later I realized the radio idea was going nowhere. I had hoped some younger people might assume the responsibility for the project, but I realized that without firm leadership the Radio Reading Service would die in its infancy. I called a second meeting and recommended we incorporate with a charter, a set of by-laws, officers and a board of directors. Everyone agreed and the group elected me president of the new organization, which allowed me to pursue the service the only way I knew how - at full speed.

I persuaded the Little Rock School Board to allow us to use their educational station KLRE as the subcarrier and then got superintendent Max Woolly to donate some space in the vocational building at the School for the Blind. Next we convinced the representatives of the various local organizations for the blind to raise $13,000 to use as seed money. With all of that in hand we had sufficient matching funds to receive a $50,000 Title XX grant through the Arkansas Department of Human Services. In March, 1981 the Arkansas Radio Reading Service made its first broadcast and by the summer was on the air eight to twelve hours a day bringing local news and other features to the visually handicapped.

Over the years the AEB has acted as an important experimental laboratory for many of the newest innovations in the rehabilitation field. Companies like to work with us because we have a larger population of blind people in a year's time than almost any place in the country. With our various overlapping programs we assist over 300 blind persons of all ages and backgrounds each year and can offer a trained professional staff to evaluate and keep comprehensive records on new devices. Just a couple of years ago the AEB tested an electronic typewriter that allowed an individual to type on a regular keyboard but produced a braille text. Recently another company devised a computer system with a magnetic card combination that functions like a talking typewriter. Through the Vocational Rehabilitation Act we have been able to purchase some of these machines to facilitate the employment of many blind individuals.

One of the problems that used to plague our program at the AEB was our inability to care for diabetics. Diabetes is one of the leading causes of blindness and yet I remember when our center hesitated to accept a diabetic because we lacked the staff to give insulin shots and conduct daily urine analysis. Over the years, primarily through research sponsored by the American Foundation for the Blind, not only have aids been developed to enable the blind diabetic to inject his own insulin but also to allow him or her to test the density of the sugar in the urine with a sound-producing instrument.

Although many of these technological devices like the Optacon, Kurzweil Reading Machine, Talking Calculator and diabetic testing equipment seem almost like magic, there is one aid that contains no sorcery at all — the use of dog guides. The modern concept of dog guides originated in the post-World War I era when the Germans begain training dogs to help blinded war veterans. An American dog breeder named Dorothy Eustis became so impressed with the work of the Germans, she founded a similar center in Morristown, New Jersey called the Seeing Eye Foundation. Since 1929, when Seeing Eye first opened, numerous other centers have appeared and by 1980 there were nine recognized schools that not only train the dogs but also train blind people to use the animals.

There is probably no symbol of the blind that is more etched in the public mind than a blind man accompanied by his dog guide. I've always found this situation a little humorous since only about three percent of America's blind population uses dog guides. Despite this fact institutions that train dogs are funded as if they had been given a license to mint money. People love dogs and people have great sympathy for the blind. The combination is irresistible and over the years some of these organizations have been able to generate surplus funds far beyond their operating costs. One director confided he could furnish a dog to every blind person that needed one from now on just on the interest accumulated from his endowments. At one point Seeing Eye wrote a letter to individuals who had contributed to the foundation in the past and asked them *not* to send any money for a while. Predictably, they received more contributions that year than they did the year before.

For the most part Seeing Eye has been generous with their funds, giving grants to other organizations, including the AEB. Nevertheless, I must confess to being a little envious of the dog schools' ability to raise money. I find it difficult to comprehend why people are willing to contribute so lavishly for a dog guide rather than to help a rehabilitation center train a blind person to have a new life. The dog centers focus only on mobility for a four-week training period. They offer no adjustment help, no braille or typing experience, no vocational counseling or training — only getting from place to place with the aid of a dog.

More often than not, the dog guide becomes another handicap to the blind individual. For example, in using a dog, dependence is merely transferred from a member of the family to an animal. There is no accompanying sense of self-confidence or independence on the part of the blind person. Also, dogs are expensive and inconvenient. They must be groomed and fed and taken on periodic visits to the veterinarian. I remember several years ago we had a vending stand operator who wanted a dog. I put him in touch with the Seeing Eye people, who trained him to use the animal. But things never worked well after he came back. During the day the poor dog had nothing to do but lie down behind the counter and on the occasions when the operator had to walk the dog around the block, the stand went unattended.

Joseph Clunk, one of the most independently mobile blind men I ever met, used to tell me how all the dog school directors wanted him to use a dog to advertise their business. He always refused, telling them, "I can't afford the contrast in intelligence. There I am going down the street and everybody says, 'Oh, look at that smart dog.'" If that didn't satisfy them, Joe would say, "Now wait a minute. I have enough trouble as it is avoiding fire plugs. I don't want to have to start looking for them."

I recall another occasion when I went to Washington, D. C. to visit Lou Rives, who was then a young attorney with the Office of Vocational Rehabilitation. He had started using a dog guide more for safety in the city than anything else. When I arrived at Lou's office everything had disappeared — his files, his furniture — everything. I crossed the hall and inquired what had happened. A young lady informed me that Lou's dog had become ill all over the office and he had taken the animal to the vet while the janitors scrubbed the floors. When I finally caught up with Lou he told me the dog was always getting sick because the secretaries and other people kept feeding the animal candy, nuts and sandwiches from their lunches, giving the dog a constant case of diarrhea. He told me the dog had created additional problems like fighting with other dogs on the street and shedding hairs on people who were allergic to dogs. On several occasions while Lou was in the midst of important conferences, he was forced to hurriedly excuse himself in order to take the dog out. The next time I saw Lou he had gone back to "independent mobility" using a cane.

From the inception of the rehabilitation center in Little Rock I opposed allowing people to bring their dogs. They could not learn independent travel as long as they relied on the dog, and with such a concentration of blind people I thought the presence of animals would be dangerous. The blind people might step on them and the dogs sometimes regard an individual with a cane as an assailant. The few times we relaxed the no-dog rule, the results always proved less than satisfactory. Once the entire women's dormitory became infested with fleas and on numerous occasions the trainees allowed their animals to defecate in the courtyard where other trainees

167

would unknowingly walk through the stuff and then track it all over the center.

In the early 1970s we did relax the no-dog rule because applicants for the taxpayer service representative program who used dog guides complained that we discriminated against them. I recognized the validity of their complaint and yielded on the issue, although I still think the presence of dogs at the center is a mistake. Because of my opposition to the dog guides, my colleagues have accused me of being a dog hater. Actually, I have always liked dogs and have always kept dogs as pets. My argument is that a blind person who is competent to undergo the necessary training to use the animal and is able to care for the daily needs of the dog is capable of learning to travel independently without the expense and other difficulties that go with the dog guide. One of the main problems is convincing people of the limitations of the dog guide. For example, it is a popular myth that dogs can distinguish the colors on traffic lights or that a blind person can start out from home and say, "Rover, take me to the office." Dogs simply cannot do these things.

I believe that everyone should have the right to choose whether or not to have a dog guide. Whenever a representative of the Seeing Eye Foundation, Leader Dogs or other dog training schools visited Little Rock, I regularly invited them to speak to our trainees because they offered a viable alternative to independent travel. I also feel strongly that every blind person should undergo training at a modern rehabilitation center first and if they cannot learn independent travel, only then should they turn to a dog guide.

Despite popular images to the contrary, dog guides are but a single innovation that has improved the quality of life for the blind over the last fifty years. The movement for agency accreditation and technologies like the Optacon and the Kurzweil Reader have also vastly accelerated the opportunities for the visually handicapped. Having witnessed the development of these devices within the span of my own lifetime, I find the prospect for even greater achievements in the 21st century to be an exciting one indeed.

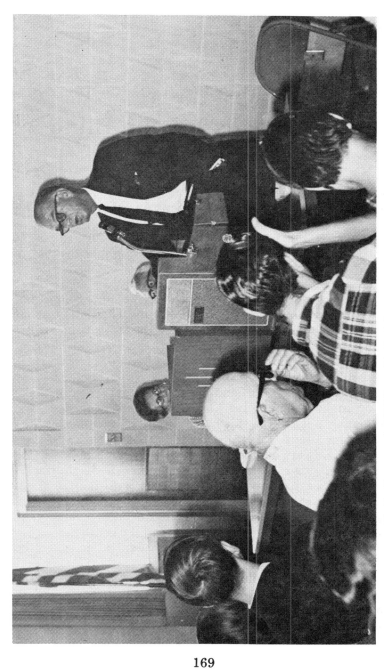

U. S. Senator J. William Fulbright was a guest speaker in 1968.

CHAPTER 11
Who Speaks for the Blind

One morning in the late 1950s, a real estate developer named Elbert Fausett telephoned me and asked if I would cut the ceremonial ribbon and make a few remarks at the opening of his newest project, the Broadmoor Shopping Center. Candidly, Fausett told me that he wanted to ask the governor to cut the ribbon, but he thought Orval Faubus might be too controversial. Fausett laughed and said he had subsequently selected me because I was the most non-controversial person he knew.

Of course, I helped Elbert open his shopping center, but his comments underscored a common misconception about those who engage in helping the blind. The truth is our work is often filled with controversy and while it is certainly a pleasant image that all blind people are a united group bound by their common handicap, this is simply a myth. In this regard, blind people are no different than their sighted counterparts. Some of the toughest competitors I know are blind people and these individuals have never shied away from a quarrel or backed down from a fight.

I have always contended that cooperation is necessary to achieve our goals. But in over forty years of rehabilitation work, I have discovered that cooperation is difficult to maintain even in the simplest of matters. Despite our common objectives, the most disruptive and bitter debates involving the work for the blind have centered around the conflict between the older established agencies and an organization called the National Federation of the Blind.

I suppose I should not have been surprised at the disruptive nature of the NFB — I had known controversy in the field long before the Federation was organized. For example, during the depression years while I was establishing the first stand program in Arkansas, the leader of a local

170

organization of blind people came to me and demanded that his group be allowed to designate each operator for the newly opened stands. When I told him the program existed for all the blind people of the state who needed employment, he became hostile and eventually launched a campaign against the program. Operating under the mistaken idea that we were in the business of giving money to the operators with no safeguards, he saw an opportunity to control enormous patronage and power. His misconceptions resulted in an ugly conflict for a while — telling blind people to stay away from the stand program, personal attacks on me through the School for the Blind alumni association, veiled threats and other disquieting measures. Eventually, he realized his campaign of harassment had been unsuccessful and the antagonism subsided. Despite combative encounters such as this one, I was unprepared for the later strife generated by the growth of the National Federation of the Blind.

The NFB originated with Jacobus ten Broek, a blind law professor at the University of California, who founded the organization in 1940. According to Frances Koestler in *The Unseen Minority*, ten Broek created the NFB to protest the "oppression of the social workers and the arrogance of the governmental administration." Twenty years later, the NFB had affiliates in forty-seven states and had been involved in several controversies and lawsuits against the established agencies and professional work for the blind. The NFB had also strongly opposed the American Association of Workers for the Blind's 1953 code of ethics because the new code condemned the practice of raising money by mailing unsolicited merchandise on a remit-or-return basis. The Federation leaders contended we aimed this section of the code directly at their major fundraising technique — the mass mailing of unordered neckties and greeting cards accompanied by a request for a donation.

By 1957 the condemnation of this practice came not only from the AAWB but from the Fraud Division of the United States Post Office as well. The postal service, according to Koestler, "charged that the letters accompanying the greeting cards falsely implied that all or most of [the money] asked for the merchandise would be used to assist the blind." In truth the NFB only received about fifteen percent of the money from

171

each sale with the remainder going to a profit-making company called Federated Industries of St. Louis. As a result of the AAWB condemnation and the post office investigation, the National Federation of the Blind became a paranoid organization — seeing enemies everywhere, especially among other groups involved in assisting the blind.

When Dr. ten Broek died in 1968, the presidency of the NFB passed to one of his most militant followers, a blind individual and outspoken former field organizer named Kenneth Jernigan. A talented and ambitious Tennessean, Jernigan held a bachelor's degree in social science from Tennessee Technological University and a master's degree in English from George Peabody College in Nashville. In 1958, Jernigan became the Director of the Iowa Commission for the Blind, which during his twenty-year tenure, he used as a base of operation for the Federation's activities.

Throughout his career, Ken Jernigan has mirrored a tremendous sense of outrage and frustration over the treatment of the blind. He blames government agencies and various private organizations for a lack of genuine advancement by blind people. He argues the significance of the fact that his group is a federation *of* the blind for *for* the blind and contends that organizations like the American Foundation for the Blind tend to be patronizing toward blind people and often contemptuous of their abilites.

Under Jernigan's leadership this attitude led the NFB into a ceaseless conflict with the National Accreditation Council. Accusing NAC of threatening the job security of blind workers and claiming that the accrediting agency wanted to destroy the NFB, the Federation launched a campaign of harassment utilizing tactics of mass protest that gained credence with other dissidents in the Vietnam era. Busing hundreds of dissatisfied blind people to NAC meetings all over the country, Jernigan used these individuals to picket meetings and divert attention from any positive activities of the national council. I first encountered one of these demonstrations at a NAC conference in Chicago in the late 1960s. Standing on the sidewalk listening to the picketers chant and shout abuse at those trying to help the blind, I realized that for the first time I felt embarrassed for my own profession. I had traveled all the way from Little Rock to work with the accrediting agency on some

172

projects I knew would benefit hundreds of visually handicapped individuals only to be met by an irrational media-oriented temper tantrum staged by a group of blind people.

Picket lines and media protests were not the only weapons in the NFB arsenal. At one point Jernigan offered to halt his harassment campaign if the board of directors of NAC revised their by-laws to allow Jernigan to name ten of the thirty-nine board members. His offer also contained the stipulation that he be allowed to remove these members if they failed to vote as he directed. At the time, I served on a committee to amend NAC's constitution and I was shocked by the number of our members who said Jernigan would destroy the accrediting agency if we did not accept his offer. I argued that if we yielded to the NFB's demands, the agency had already been destroyed.

By a narrow vote we rejected Jernigan's proposal. We did, however, invite the Federation and other consumer-oriented groups to submit a list of people they would like to see on the board and we would consider them. But Jernigan rejected this counteroffer and by refusing to allow any of his membership to serve on our board, he closed any possible avenue of constructive communication.

Unable to stop NAC or dominate its board, Jernigan and the NFB attempted to seize control of other organizations. In the late 1970s these efforts led to a struggle for control of the prestigious Minneapolis Society for the Blind, one of the oldest agencies in the midwest. Founded around the turn of the century as a workshop and home for the blind the Minneapolis Society had later expanded its facilities to include a modern rehabilitation center. The original charter of the organization provided that anyone who paid the one-dollar membership fee had a vote in selecting the Society's board of directors. The Federation discovered this clause and set out to dominate the organization by having all Federation members throughout the country join the Minneapolis Society and then elect an all-NFB board.

The Society took the matter to court, but the local judge ruled that the charter provision had to stand. The result was a "battle of the ballots" between the NFB and concerned workers for the blind throughout the nation.

173

In Arkansas I presented the situation to the board of the Arkansas Enterprises for the Blind, and each member responded by donating a dollar to join the Minneapolis Society and signing a proxy to vote for the slate of officers that opposed the takeover by the NFB. Although I managed to get over a hundred people in Arkansas to join the Minneapolis Society, I had little hope of defeating the organized efforts of a nation-wide group like the Federation. Our cause seemed especially hopeless since Ken Jernigan boasted that the NFB's secret membership list contained 50,000 names.

Several weeks later I received a jubilant phone call from an old friend who served on the board of the Minneapolis Society. In the results of the election announced that morning, the NFB had only been able to muster 12,000 votes and their candidates had lost by almost 5,000 votes. Jernigan's claim of 50,000 members appeared to have been nothing but a bluff and I regarded the whole affair as a great victory over the disruptive tactics of the Federation.

Over the years I often wished it had been possible for me to view the activities of the NFB with nothing but concerned detachment — a distant observer of battles such as the one in Minneapolis. Unfortunately, I never had that opportunity. Beginning in the mid-1950s, the Federation selected Arkansas as a target area and this decision in turn thrust me into the center of one of the most bitter controversies of my career.

I first heard about the NFB during the Second World War when a member of our alumni association, who had recently returned from a trip to California, suggested we affiliate with this new group. Joe Clunk happened to be in Little Rock at the time and I asked if he knew anything about the Federation. I remember his voice took on a serious edge as he advised me not to get involved with the NFB because the main thrust of their group centered on opposition to all professional work for the blind. After I explained this to our membership we almost unanimously voted down the motion to join the Federation.

A few years later, as I became involved in the national politics of the AAWB, I heard more and more about the Federation and its activities. The NFB leadership constantly attacked the American Foundation for the Blind and other established agencies. Claiming they were run by sighted people who did not understand the problems of the blind, the

174

Federation representatives accused these organizations of being patronizing and actually hindering blind people from making real progress. Since I vehemently disagreed with this position I was delighted when, in 1951, I received an invitation to participate on a panel in response to a speech by Jacobus ten Broek at the annual convention of the National Rehabilitation Association at Los Angeles.

The panel included the executive director of the AFB and the Chief of Services for the Blind in Washington. The participation of these men indicated that Jacobus ten Broek had definitely made waves among those concerned with the welfare of the blind.

Almost as soon as Dr. ten Broek began his talk I realized why he drew so much attention. He was a consummate showman — a deep resonant voice, a full beard and a set of braille notes which he tossed page by page on the floor with a grand flourish as he finished each one. The essence of his message was that everything being done by the establishment actually harmed visually handicapped persons and only the organized blind knew what was best for the blind. He contended blind people should control their own destiny without the interference of patronizing sighted individuals and he castigated those who had led the blind to this present state of dependence.

I found ten Broek's speech disturbing. In all my years of work with the visually handicapped in Arkansas I had experienced great success with an approach based on teamwork and cooperation between the blind and the sighted. I could see no advantage to the blind in rejecting the help of their many friends who could see. After the meeting I spoke with Dr. ten Broek and tried to convince him we all shared a common goal — to achieve better opportunities for all blind people. I suggested we exchange ideas and seek some common ground rather than continuing the existing state of hostilities. I finally invited him to address the AAWB convention the next year in Louisville and offered to speak to the NFB convention in Nashville to explain the goals of our organization. After the uncompromising militancy of his speech, he surprised me by eagerly accepting my offer.

A year later, despite some opposition from our program committee, I scheduled Dr. ten Broek to address a morning session at the Louisville conference. The panel chairman explained that each of our three speakers would be alloted fifteen minutes and then we would have a period for questions. Dr. ten Broek spoke first and gave a similar performance to the one I witnessed in Los Angeles. After about twenty minutes, however, the chairman interrupted him and said, "I'm sorry, Dr. ten Broek, but we have other panelists and I thought you understood the speeches would only be for fifteen minutes."

The Federation president turned to him and growled, "I see what you're doing. When I get to the part of my talk that hurts a little, you cut me off. Right?"

To my chagrin the audience began applauding and cheering Dr. ten Broek. Our disconcerted chairman asked for order and replied, "Well all right, I will defer to the audience. Do you want to hear more of Dr. ten Broek's speech?" The crowd burst into wild and enthusiastic applause.

Seated on the platform, I observed these proceedings in a state of total surprise. I could not understand what had happened. The Federation president spoke for another twenty minutes and the other speakers were reduced to a few moments each. Later that day I did some investigating and discovered that ten Broek had quietly and deliberately infiltrated the audience with loyal NFB members. The Federation leadership had planned and rehearsed the whole performance, using our hospitality to create a false impression of support for their point of view.

Dr. ten Broek's deception angered our members and several people urged me not to attend the NFB meeting in Nashville. While I felt betrayed, I also believed it would serve no positive purpose to fail to fulfill my part of our bargain.

The next morning I invited Dr. ten Broek to join me for breakfast in my hotel room. I still hoped to establish a line of communication and I found him to be a likeable individual when he was not playing to the crowd. We discussed several matters and after a while I asked him, "Why do you insist on doing things this way? Making everything so antagonistic. Surrounding yourself with controversy. You have an important position at the university. There should be no need for such bitterness."

Dr. ten Broek surprised me with an amazingly candid answer. There was no long-winded harangue, no soapbox political speech. Instead, he told me about his personal disappointments within the legal profession. He felt he was not recognized for his own ability by many of his colleagues and indicated he might have been the dean of the law school if he had been a sighted professor.

I realized then that in many ways the Federation represented the extension of one blind man's lifelong frustration and hostility — blaming society for their handicap; withdrawing to a point where only the blind could understand their hurt; distrusting everyone else. Consequently, my breakfast meeting strengthened my resolve to address the NFB meeting in Nashville.

Two weeks later I spoke to a session of the Federation's convention at the stately old Andrew Jackson Hotel. In my remarks I stressed the theme of teamwork — the things that might be achieved through the cooperation of the blind, the local community, and state and federal agencies. Although some of my friends in the AAWB had warned me, the barrage of catcalls, boos and general heckling that greeted my speech appalled me. The members of the Federation refused to listen to another point of view. Following the meeting I packed my bags and returned to Little Rock, saddened that there seemed to be no sense of shared objectives between the NFB and the other agencies dedicated to helping the blind. Unfortunately, I had to go back to Arkansas to discover how wide this breach had become.

Several weeks after the Nashville fiasco, an NFB organizer named George Card appeared in Little Rock and began efforts to form a Federation chapter. Focusing his recruiting efforts on the more than thirty stand operators throughout the state, Card promised these people that if they joined the NFB, the organization would restructure the program so they could own their own stands. Card also promised several of them what I regarded as "pie-in-the-sky" ideas based on the philosophy that society can never pay a sufficient debt to the blind. But since the operators already had their own association, Card failed to convince enough people to shift to the Federation.

Card had more success with the Arkansas Braille Club, a social organization designed to give the blind a sense of belonging and to provide a program of organized recreation.

At the time George Card visited Arkansas, the president of the group was an old school friend of mine named Ray Penix. Ray had been the first blind person to graduate from the University of Arkansas and although he had considerable ability, had never been able to find his niche in life. He graduated with a degree in music, but he had tried a variety of things like teaching at the School for the Blind, running a legitimate massage parlor, chiropratic school and a few other endeavors. The ideas of the NFB excited Ray to the point that he invited Jacobus ten Broek to travel to Arkansas and speak to the Braille Club. Since I had to be out of town when Dr. ten Broek spoke, several friends of mine attended and reported that the Federation president delivered a scathing attack on me, on the rehabilitation center and on the state agency people who worked directly with the blind.

Dr. ten Broek also proposed that the members of the Braille Club vote to affiliate their organization with the NFB. I felt somewhat vindicated when the membership voted this proposition down because Penix and ten Broek told them they would have to amend our constitution to prohibit any sighted people from holding office. To their credit, my friends in the Braille Club had always had a good relationship with their sighted members and saw no need to close the door on them.

Ray Penix's experience with the Federation was like a religious conversion. He resigned from the Braille Club and recruited enough people to found the first chapter of the NFB in Arkansas. Once established, the local chapter then devoted a tremendous amount of effort to discrediting the AEB rehabilitation center in Little Rock. In Louisiana, for example, they discovered that the state had spent over $200,000 in rehabilitation fees for instruction in Little Rock. Louisiana Federation members went to their state legislature and told the legislators that they were wasting their rehabilitation money and should keep those funds in their own state. The NFB even started spreading rumors to the effect that we used drugs at the center and that I had become wealthy by exploiting the blind people of Louisiana and other states.

I finally confronted Ray and asked him what he wanted. When he indicated he wanted my job, I told him there was no guarantee the center's board would select him even if I resigned (which I had no intention of doing). He said that even if he failed to get the job, the Federation would bring someone from out of state to do it. "Roy, don't you see?" he pleaded. "It's for the good of the Federation." I stopped myself from asking Ray about the good of the blind people we had been serving for so long and let the matter drop. It served no purpose to argue with a fanatic who had lost sight of our basic goals.

By the mid-1950s my problems with the Federation came not only from the local group but from the national organization as well. Over the years the NFB had devised a scheme of getting into a state for the purpose of organizing and recruiting members and at the same time attacking the existing agencies for the blind. They would offer to conduct a free survey of the various services for the blind in the state and then make recommendations for improvements in the quality and efficiency of those services. These surveys gave the Federation a respectability the organization would not ordinarily have received.

Early in 1955 I received a letter from Arkansas' new governor, Orval Faubus, informing me that a team from the National Federation of the Blind would soon be in Little Rock to begin such a survey. I had never met the governor, but I did know his executive secretary, Arnold Sikes. Arnold had been a young county clerk when we opened a vending stand in Paris, Arkansas and I phoned him to find out why the governor had turned to the NFB. He told me that Ray Penix recommended the survey to Faubus as an inexpensive way to help the blind and since Ray's uncle, state senator Roy Milum, supported Faubus, the governor had agreed to the project. Arnold also informed me that since our center was not a state agency we were not obligated to cooperate with the survey.

Choosing my words carefully, I told Arnold that the NFB had no interest in improving services for the blind. Rather, they only wanted to attack existing organizations and recruit disgruntled blind people into their ranks. I pointed out that the organization's activities could be harmful if the Federation destroyed the confidence of a large number of blind people in the local agencies that served them.

Following my discussion with Arnold Sikes, I wrote a personal letter to Governor Faubus. I informed the governor that based on professional ethics, I could not recognize the Federation team as being professionally competent to evaluate

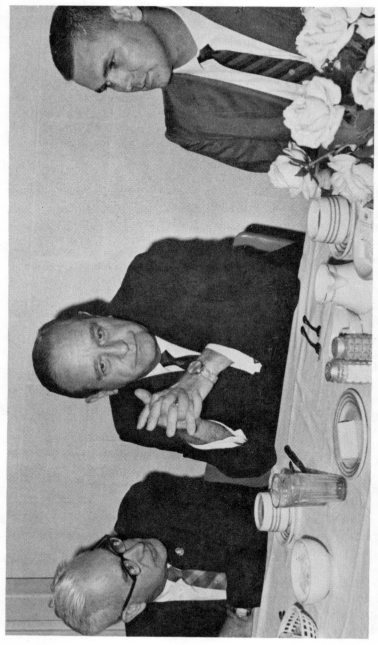

Arkansas Governor Orval Faubus was a guest speaker for a trainee banquet in the early 1960's.

our program at the center. In the concluding paragraph of that letter I commended Faubus for his interest in the blind, but also recommended he utilize the services of the American Foundation for the Blind or the federal Office of Rehabilitation to conduct the needed survey.

A few weeks later Lila Lampkin telephoned me at home and told me to turn my radio to a local talk show. The program featured a representative of the NFB and as the show progressed, he made all kinds of wild assertions — giving the Federation sole credit for the Randolph-Sheppard Act, claiming the Federation was the only responsible organization working to help the blind, saying the state agencies exploited the blind. I could not believe these people would issue a stream of falsehoods like that on the public airways. But the worst came later. The survey team called on the Director of Rehabilitation and demanded access to confidential records. When the director refused, they approached the governor and demanded the director be fired.

George Card and Kenneth Jernigan, the same individual who would later be president of the organization, headed the NFB survey team. Despite my own misgivings, I tried to be cordial to them when they arrived to inspect the rehabilitation center. I told them I had no objections to their examining our facilities, but I wanted them to understand my position. Then I had Lila read them the letter I had earlier written to the governor. Card and Jernigan became so furious they stormed out of the center without completing their survey.

This anger surfaced again when they released their final report of eighty pages of mimeographed material with almost a quarter of it devoted to personal attacks on me. They charged I had been a dictator in the vending stand program and had used my position to punish blind people who would not conform to my dictates. The report also implied that during the war, $10,000 had mysteriously disappeared from the agency.

A reporter for the *Arkansas Gazette*, the state's largest newspaper, telephoned me for a reaction to the report. I had known him since my city council days and I felt relaxed in talking with him. I gave him some background on the Federation and in the course of our conversation said, "Well, they [the NFB] are just another vicious and unscrupulous pressure group." The story that appeared in the paper contained that

181

statement and although I suspected the quote might cause trouble later on, by that time I had more serious matters on my mind.

The Federation spent hundreds of dollars to distribute its report. Using a mass mailing technique, they circulated the document all over the state to lawyers, doctors, state legislators, librarians and to anyone they felt might influence the direction of the work for the blind in Arkansas. At first I didn't think anyone would pay attention to the report, but one day my brother-in-law stopped by our house to recount a conversation he had overheard in a local drugstore. A Little Rock physician had asked his companions if any of them had ever heard of Roy Kumpe. "Well, he's a terrible individual," the doctor had said. "He's exploiting the blind. I just got this report in the mail — it was written by some concerned blind people — and I tell you, something ought to be done about this Kumpe fellow."

I realized then that some people were paying attention to the report; a document that libeled me and discredited my life's work. After a brief period in which I was almost unable to comprehend that this kind of sordid activity could be a part of the work for the blind, I received another shock — a U. S. marshal presented me with a summons containing the information that I was being sued for $250,000 by Kenneth Jernigan, George Card and Jacobus ten Broek. They were also suing the *Arkansas Gazette* for the same amount contending my earlier comments in the newspaper had libeled their organization.

This news quickly turned my sadness into anger. I contacted my old friend and attorney, William Nash, who reminded me there are only three defenses to a libel suit. First, that you did not say it; second, you said it and they weren't damaged; and third, you said it and it was the truth. After reading the NFB report, Nash advised me to file a counter-suit for $250,000 since I had been libeled and not the other way around.

After filing my own suit, the proceedings dragged on for over a year. This was a difficult time, not just for me, but for my family as well. I vividly recall one evening when my younger son Peter said, "Daddy, why are the blind people against you when you work for the blind?"

182

Comments like this plus the general tension of the situation cast a gray cloud over my life for quite some time. Ironically, Governor Faubus aided my cause when he publicly condemned the Federation's survey, saying it had been used as the basis for a membership drive among the blind people of the state. I also felt gratified when the governor said he was dissatisfied with the final report because it "failed to acknowledge the wonderful work of the Lions Clubs of Arkansas in their support of the AEB Rehabilitation Center at Little Rock." Finally, Faubus concluded his remarks on the matter by observing that the Federation's report included personal criticisms "which should not be included in a document of this kind."

After an agonizingly long period of time the NFB sent word to the *Gazette's* attorney that if I would drop my suit, they would drop theirs. I had mixed feelings about the offer. On the one hand I wanted to fight them to the end and expose them for what they were. But our board of directors wanted to drop the matter and I partially agreed with their argument that we should not be in the position of publicly fighting other blind organizations. I had to keep in mind that the Federation represented a small minority and I needed to concentrate my efforts on the blind people that we helped every day at the rehabilitation center. Thus the law suits were quietly dropped on both sides.

About a decade later while attending a conference in New York, Ken Jernigan called on me in my hotel room. We chatted amiably for a while and then Jernigan said, "Roy, I don't know how to say this, but I want to apologize for what I did back there in Arkansas ten years ago. I guess the only excuse is that I was young and inexperienced." Human beings are complex creatures and Ken Jernigan is perhaps more complex than most. I regarded his apology as a decent gesture and accepted it as such. But because of our divergent philosophies, I knew there would be future confrontations between the Federation and myself and sadly enough, events proved me right.

The controversies in Arkansas between the Federation and established agencies continued into the 1970s. In 1975 NAC officials selected Little Rock as the site of the annual National Accreditation Council meeting. As chairman of the host committee, I devoted several weeks to preparing for the meeting at the Camelot Inn, the city's new convention facility. I knew it was no coincidence that the state chapter of the NFB scheduled its own meeting the same week down the street at the Holiday Inn, but I tried to ignore this situation and hoped for the best.

November 12, 1975 dawned in a cold and hazy fog and the bleakness of the weather only intensified my apprehensive mood. During a breakfast meeting in conjunction with the NAC conference, Anna New, a NAC staff member from New York, hurried into the dining room and announced, "They're on their way." Everyone in the room knew what she meant.

Outside, almost one hundred sign-carrying blind individuals had braved the chilly weather and marched the six blocks from the Holiday Inn to the Camelot. They formed a long picket line in front of our hotel as they brandished signs with messages like "NAC is a Pain" and "We Can Speak for Ourselves." The local television cameras recorded the whole scene — the drama of the blind struggling against the blind. I went outside and overheard a NFB spokesman being interviewed by a television reporter. "We've tracked NAC across the country," the Federation representative said. "And we know that NAC will have to be destroyed because it refuses to be reformed." "Because it refused to do what we say" was what he should have said.

I felt particularly hurt by the demonstration. Not only because the whole spectacle took place in Little Rock but also because several of our local blind people played prominent roles in the exhibition. Some of these individuals had gone through our program at the center and I knew and liked many of them. It distressed me to see them turn to such counter-productive and radical extremes to try and solve their problems.

Because the AEB had received accreditation from NAC, some of the Federation decided to temporarily abandon the hotel and picket the center. Before they arrived I received a call from one of our former trainees, a young man from another state who worked in the vending stand program there. That morning he telephoned to say hello, but when I found out his trip had been sponsored by the Federation, I became cautious and asked, "Were you in that picket line yesterday at the Camelot?"

184

He laughed and replied, "No, I started out with them, but all those damn fools wanted to do was march around in the cold and chant and wave their signs. I just came down for the bus ride."

"Are you coming out to picket the center?" I queried.

"Oh hell no, Mr. Kumpe, you know me better than that. Beside, I hooked up with this gal on the bus and we've made other plans. All this is nothing but a free vacation — free bus ride, free hotel, free meals, and free whiskey."

The whole conversation lightened my spirits. Not that I didn't take the Federation seriously, but my talk with that young man did show me a lighter side of a grim situation.

The Federation leadership argues that blindness is an attitude. The blind are not truly handicapped, only inconvenienced. They contend that our biggest hurdle is changing the attitude of the sighted community, for when their attitudes change then we will all be equal. The fact is, there is no way blind individuals and sighted individuals can be equal unless in the words of Lou Rives "we can restore the sight of all blind people or put out the eyes of all sighted people." Blindness is more than an attitude problem and blind people are foolish to reject all help from their sighted friends.

The NFB has never been approved by the Better Business Bureau or the National Information Bureau because the Federation's leadership refuses to publicly reveal the group's financial records. The organization's main goal has always been to dominate and control all work for the blind. Thus, over the last three decades the Federation has opposed virtually every progressive step for the blind. Far too often their ridiculous charges and accusations have served to undermine the confidence blind people have in the very agencies that are doing the most to serve them. The NFB contends all established agencies harm the blind. But what do they offer as an alternative to these organizations? Very, very little. Over the last forty years I have met hundreds of people, blind and sighted, who with a crusader-like zeal have devoted their lives to furthering opportunities for the blind and improving the general welfare of the visually handicapped. I refuse to believe that all of these people have been malevolent empire builders as the Federation implies.

Fortunately, there are two consumer-oriented groups that have embraced a different philosophy from that of the NFB. The first of these organizations is the American Council of the Blind. The ACB actually resulted from a schism within the ranks of the Federation. In 1961 Dr. ten Broek expelled several state affiliates that had opposed his leadership of the NFB. Under the direction of Durwood McDaniels, a blind attorney from Oklahoma City, and several other individuals the expelled Federation chapters formed the American Council of the Blind. From my perspective, one of the ironies of the division was that my old antagonist, George Card, was one of the ejected Federation members who joined the newly formed Council.

For several years the ACB has advocated working through the established agencies to improve services for the blind. Larger than the Federation, the American Council of the Blind is a more democratic organization and has become a respected spokesman for the needs of the visually handicapped.

The second group is the Blinded Veterans Association. Like the Council, the BVA works closely with other agencies and supports the work of the National Accreditation Council with representation on the board. In contrast to the antagonistic approach of the Federation, these two organizations have demonstrated the effectiveness of mutual assistance and teamwork in helping blind persons achieve their individual goals.

Our aim is to help the blind. The way to achieve that objective is through cooperation. Unquestionably, there are differences of opinion and this is as it should be. But the resolution of these differences should be through debate and dialogue, not through picket lines and character assassination. Almost fifty years ago my colleague Leonard Robinson, while campaigning for the Randolph-Sheppard Act, summed up my own sentiments when he said, "The first thing which the agencies for the blind can do for the blind is to forget their petty jealousies of each other and learn to cooperate with one another more harmoniously to the best interests of the blind." Maybe someday we can all make Leonard's hope a reality.

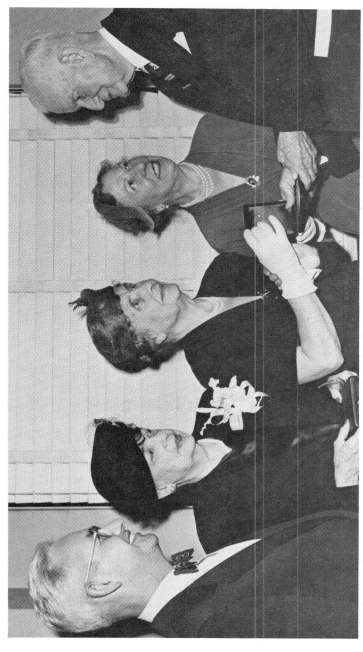

During Foundation Day, 1952, at the American Foundation for the Blind, Roy Kumpe, Daisy Rogers, Helen Keller and Polly Thompson presented the Migel Medal to T. J. Watson, Sr., president of IBM.

CHAPTER 12
Reflections

In over forty years of working with the visually handicapped, my theme has always been that blindness is no respecter of persons. Loss of sight affects wealthy people as well as the poor, youngsters as well as the aged, the highly educated as well as the illiterate. Blindness strikes individuals regardless of nationality, religion or race. When we founded the rehabilitation center in Arkansas, I knew we would have to serve clients on a regional basis and I suspected that someday we would offer our services to trainees on a nationwide scale. But in the beginning, I never dreamed that eventually our program would become international in scope.

As various individuals visited the AEB under the sponsorship of the United Nations or the U.S. State Department, I became interested in their respective countries and how each of these nations dealt with the problems of blindness. Since the Lions are an international organization, I not only wanted to expand our services to meet the needs of blind people from foreign countries, but I also wanted to journey to those nations and observe the kinds of assistance being offered citizens with visual handicaps. As a result, over the last two decades, many of my fondest memories center around our foreign trainees and the many places all over the world in which I have had the opportunity to travel.

Our first international trainee, Yong Bong Park of Seoul, South Korea, came to the center following the Korean War. Although awarded a scholarship to Perkins School for the Blind in Watertown, Massachusetts, Mr. Park decided to follow the recommendation of Tuk Heung Lee, the superintendent of Korea's National School for the Blind, and participate in our adjustment program before proceeding to Massachusetts. Since the AEB was being asked to provide free training, I had

188

to propose the idea to our board. At first some board members hesitated because we were operating on a limited budget, but I convinced them the training of a foreign national would be both a challenge and an opportunity.

Even though Mr. Park had a college degree in English literature when he arrived at the center, language proved to be a formidable obstacle since English with a Korean accent widely differs from English with an Arkansas accent. Once we overcame this initial barrier, Mr. Park learned mobility and the other basic skills we taught and became one of our most beloved trainees. After three months at the AEB he proceeded to Boston to accept his scholarship at Perkins. Before completing his nine-month tenure in the east, Mr. Park wrote me and asked if he could spend another summer at the AEB before returning to Korea. Because his first visit with us had been so successful, our board agreed to this extension and Mr. Park spent an additional three months in Little Rock.

Upon returning to Seoul, Mr. Park worked as an instructor at the local school for the blind before founding the first rehabilitation center for the adult blind in the history of Korea. With the aid of an ophthalmologist, he established a training program that included orientation and mobility instruction, braille, and personal adjustment training. Mr. Park and his wife founded a braille publication in an effort to create a sense of community among the blind of Korea. In the early 1960s he wrote me that he had been named the executive director of the Korean National Council for the Blind, which coordinated all of the work for the visually handicapped throughout the nation.

In 1979 Berenice and I had the opportunity to tour East Asia and our trip included a lengthy visit with Mr. Park and his wife in Seoul. I was amazed at what this man had accomplished with the minimal instruction he had received in the United States. Because of financial pressures, Mr. Park had been unable to earn a living for his family from the rehabilitation center, so he had worked as a masseur at night. In Korea, only blind persons are trained and licensed in this area and even though his wife objected to his being a masseur because of his high level of education, Mr. Park found that this was the only way he could earn enough money to support himself while he kept the center open. Blessed with a great deal of imagination and energy, eventually Mr. Park opened his own massage clinic and hired other blind individuals to work for him. In Korea, hotels offer massage as a basic service like a barbershop or beauty shop and the blind of Korea regarded our host as a successful and wealthy person.

During our stay in Seoul, Mr. Park arranged for us to use a car with a driver to explore the city and held a banquet dinner in our honor. We thoroughly enjoyed the reunion and greatly admired Mr. Park's fine work for the blind in Korea.

Although we have trained numerous individuals from East Asia, along with Yong Bong Park, a young Korean girl named Kim Wickes made a special impression on me. During the North Korean invasion of the south in 1950, Kim and her family lost their home and became refugees, fleeing before the invading army. At one point, despite warnings not to look, three-year-old Kim watched the explosion of a bomb that detonated near the family. The flash scarred the corneas of her eyes and left the little girl totally blind.

A few days later Kim's father became so despondent over the hopeless situation, he threw Kim and her two-year-old sister into a nearby river in a misguided effort to save his children from more misery. His wife's pleas caused him to reverse his irrational decision and although he rescued Kim, the other child drowned.

The family rejoined the other refugees and walked over two hundred miles to the southern tip of South Korea. During the arduous journey, the mother became separated from the rest of the family and again in desperation, Kim's father placed his remaining daughter in an orphanage and then disappeared.

Kim spent seven years as the only blind child in the Christian Missionary Orphanage until a family named Wickes from Indianapolis, Indiana heard about her though an international relief agency and adopted her. The Wickes put their new daughter through the Indiana School for the Blind and then through Wheaton Academy and the University of Indiana, where she majored in music.

Because of her musical talent and academic ability, Kim received a Fulbright Scholarship to study music in Vienna. During her residence in Austria she participated in a series of religious musical festivals in Switzerland. While performing

190

at one of these events, Kim met the American evangelist Billy Graham, who invited her to sing with his religious crusade.

After working with Graham for a while, Kim moved to West Memphis, Arkansas, where she started her own ministry under the sponsorship of some local businessmen. Soon afterwards, I invited her to come to Little Rock to address one of our monthly luncheons because I knew what a tremendous inspiration she would be to our trainees. Her performance more than exceeded my expectations. Accompanied by recorded music, she illustrated her talk with several beautiful songs and left everyone at the AEB talking about her visit for weeks.

After the luncheon, I escorted Kim on a tour of the center. During our conversation she said, "Oh my, I wish I had known about a rehabilitation program like this. I never had the opportunity to learn some of these things."

Kim impressed me so much that I invited her to sing for our upcoming Visiting District Governors' Day and in exchange offered her the chance to train at the center for a while. She accepted my proposal and spent a few weeks with us, allowing the AEB to claim her as a former trainee. Over the last few years, I have tried to help her ministry by recommending her to various religious and civic groups. I think she has a wonderful and inspirational message and I also believe she represents what a talented and determined blind person can accomplish.

As I became more enthusiastic about training people from other countries at the center, I began to realize there were many inherent difficulties in this type of expansion. With an increasing number of foreign applications we needed additional funds since the tuition and training fees for these people could not be paid by a state vocational rehabilitation agency. I also perceived a reluctance on the part of some of the local Lions Club members to share our limited funds with people from other countries. To overcome these obstacles, I approached several internationally oriented foundations about possible grants to help offset the cost of training foreign nationals.

I soon discovered that when I mentioned the Arkansas Enterprises for the Blind, foundation directors, especially those in the east, immediately lost interest in my proposal. They assumed any institution in Arkansas would be limited in scope and thought the word "Enterprises" connoted a workshop. In their minds, a struggling workshop in the backwoods of Arkansas deserved little, if any, consideration for a grant to train blind people from all over the world.

Out of frustration we considered changing the name of the center, but because of state pride, most of our board members resisted this move. To solve the dilemma, I suggested the AEB incorporate another organization with a separate and more international name that would act as an affiliate service.

As a result, in 1971 we incorporated the International Services for the Blind. The ISB functioned as both a fund-raising organization and one that sponsored research and the training of professional men and women from various nations in response to a world-wide demand for increased rehabilitation services for the blind. Soon after its inauguration, our new organization received recognition and assistance from a variety of groups including the Partners of the Americas, Lions International Foundation, Rotary International and the Pan American Health Organization. The first line of support for the ISB, however, soon became our own annual light bulb sale. Through an agreement with Westinghouse, we acted as a broker for selling light bulbs to Lions Clubs and other civic groups for their individual fundraising efforts. This undertaking gave us a regular source of funds for the international program.

The ISB proved to be a successful venture from the beginning and in 1974 the World Council for the Welfare of the Blind accepted our organization as a voting member. Over the years we have maintained the ISB as a separate non-profit group that contracts for management and other services with the Arkansas Enterprises for the Blind. As the Executive Director of the AEB, I coordinated the work of the International Services for the Blind and upon my retirement the board elected me to serve as the president of the ISB on a volunteer basis. The ISB board meets annually and reflects a global character with members from Mexico City, Colombia, and Saudi Arabia, as well as the United States.

Over the past few years my work with the ISB has broadened my awareness of the discrepancies that exist from nation to nation in regard to the work for the blind. While some countries offer advanced and sophisticated new systems to aid

192

their blind citizens, other nations lag decades behind in providing any kind of assistance for visually handicapped adults.

While my duties with the ISB have increased my understanding of these differences, my own personal travels have provided me with firsthand knowledge of exactly how the movement for the blind is progressing throughout the world.

My first foreign venture took place under the auspices of the American Foundation for the Overseas Blind, when a representative of that organization asked me to take a short-term assignment as a consultant in El Salvador in 1963. Since I had always been interested in travel as well as the international character of the work for the blind, I eagerly accepted the invitation.

Accompanied by Berenice and our younger son, Peter, I spent six weeks in El Salvador helping to expand a school for blind children to include a rehabilitation program for blind adults. During our stay we lived on the campus and made a host of friends among the students and staff. The school's physical plant consisted of a million-dollar facility donated by one of the country's wealthiest families. In fact, several wealthy individuals enhanced the institution's program by volunteering on a regular basis. An American-educated ophthalmologist served as the official director of the program, although a young lady named Irma Gomez ran the day-to-day operation of the school.

The state had earlier organized a Commission for the Handicapped which aided the volunteer group with the funding of their program and I felt that, at that time, the officials of El Salvador had made a fine start in their overall program to aid the blind and other handicapped persons. In my final report I recommended the agency maintain the rehabilitation center for the adult blind and consider placing some of their "graduates" in assembly-line jobs. I toured a local cigarette factory and identified some positions that could easily be filled by blind workers.

Before we left El Salvador, I invited Irma Gomez to come to the United States and visit our center in Little Rock and a few years later she accepted my offer. Irma studied Arkansas's vending stand program closely and when she returned to El Salvador she initiated a project to establish stand locations for

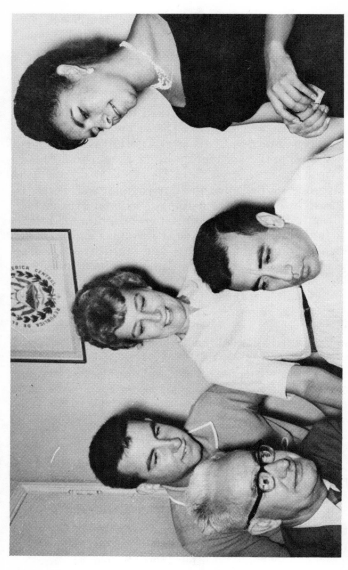

Roy Kumpe served as a technical consultant to the government of El Salvador in 1963. Pictured are (seated) Kumpe and Dr. Anturo Carlos Flores. In the background are (from left) Peter Kumpe, Berenice Kumpe and Irma Gomez.

blind persons in her own country. She did a remarkable job of following through on our recommendations and had a real impact on improving the services for the blind in El Salvador. From time to time, under the auspices of the ISB, she sent a few of her staff members to Little Rock for further training at our center.

I have never met anyone more dedicated to serving the blind than Irma Gomez. For twenty years she lived at the school, devoting her life to aiding the blind individuals who came to the facility for aid. The last time I saw Irma at a conference in 1979, she seemed under tremendous stress. The Marxist terrorists of El Salvador had launched a prerevolutionary campaign of assassination and intimidation and she told us that she often found hastily scrawled bomb threats lying on her desk or tacked to the door of her office.

She had adopted a little girl and just before Christmas in 1980 we received a letter from Irma saying that conditions had degenerated to a point that she had resigned her position at the school to go into hiding because of personal threats to herself and her child. That message was the last communication I received from Irma and every time I remember her I am reminded of the tragedy of this dedicated woman whose dreams of a lifetime were destroyed by political fanaticism.

Long before my trip to El Salvador and my friendship with Irma, I met a fascinating visually handicapped young man from Bogota, Colombia. A graduate student at George Peabody College for Teachers in Nashville, Tennessee, Hernando Pradilla visited our rehabilitation center in Little Rock during his Thanksgiving vacation in 1953. Because he admired our program I invited him to return and be our guest for a month after his graduation. He accepted my offer and became so inspired by our work at the AEB that when he returned to Bogota, he secured the cooperation of the Lions and other groups to establish his own rehabilitation center based on the model of the Arkansas Enterprises for the Blind.

Along the way, as we instructed several additional foreign trainees, the American Foundation for Overseas Blind (now Helen Keller International) recognized our work and began to refer other individuals from abroad to the AEB for training. For example, they sent Homero de Gregorio to Little Rock for his initial adjustment training. A middle-aged man from

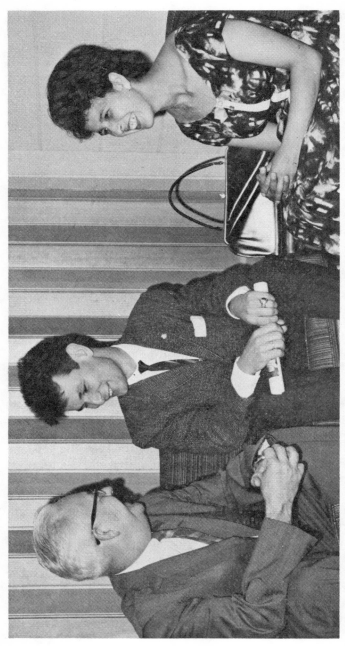

One of AEB's early international trainees was Hernando Pradilla, who returned to his native Bogota, Colombia and established a rehabilitation center modeled after AEB. Pictured with Kumpe and Pradilla during a 1964 visit to AEB is Mrs. Pradilla.

Montevideo, Uruguay, Homero had been a businessman and a member of the Lions Club before losing his sight. Like Hernando Pradilla, Homero completed our course, returned to his native land and started a rehabilitation center for blind adults. We had a similar experience with Matthew Mussa, a young man who trained at the AEB and then went home to Panama City, Panama to develop a rehabilitation facility in cooperation with the Salvation Army.

Some of the proudest moments in my career came in 1971 when I toured the rehabilitation centers of Hernando Pradilla, Homero de Gregorio, Irma Gomez and Matthew Mussa in Latin America. To find each one of these former AEB trainees at the forefront of his respective nation's attempts to aid the blind gave me the gratifying sensation that my own life's work had made an impact on the international movement to help the visually handicapped.

Despite the fine efforts of these AEB alumni, the attitudes toward blindness in most Latin American nations continue to lag behind the United States by as much as fifty years. On our tour in 1971 we talked to many people who still believed that if a person went blind they were automatically condemned to a life of idleness. If that sightless individual came from an affluent family, he or she would be cared for, but if they lived in poverty, they would be forced to beg on the streets for the remainder of their lives. I remembered the many people in Arkansas who held similar beliefs a half century earlier and I recalled the struggles we went through to change those attitudes. I can only hope that my friends helping the blind in Latin America will be able to destroy those misconceptions faster than we did in some parts of the United States.

The year after my Latin American journey, I attended the International Rehabilitation Congress in Sydney, Australia. While I enjoyed the Congress itself as an informative international exchange of ideas and an opportunity to renew old friendships, on a side trip to New Zealand I discovered the most comprehensive program for the blind I have observed anywhere in the world. If the attitudes toward the blind in Latin America reflected the past, the programs in New Zealand provided a vision of the future.

The New Zealand Foundation for the Blind started as a volunteer organization in the 1880s. Later, when the government became involved in various social welfare programs, officials continued to operate in the area of aid for the blind under a contractual agreement with the private organization rather than establish a purely state-operated system.

As one counselor told me, New Zealand's goal is to serve the blind from "womb to tomb." This comprehensive program includes an ultra modern school for the blind, an eye care and blindness prevention program subsidized by the state and a sytem of hostelries or homes for the elderly blind which are pleasant places operated in a manner designed to maintain the dignity of the individual.

The New Zealanders also finance the college educations of qualified blind persons and even have a governmental system to pay for special teachers for blind youngsters who choose to remain in public school rather than the national residential school for the blind. Perhaps the most amazing facet of the plan involves placing every blind person in New Zealand on a computer register. Each individual on that list receives a visit once a year by a field staff member of the agency or a social worker and in addition receives a monthly pension regardless of their economic status.

While the population of New Zealand is relatively small with a limited number of blind people, nevertheless, no other country offers such a comprehensive program to help their visually handicapped citizens. The New Zealand system offers the rest of the world a magnificent model of progressive attitudes toward aiding the blind.

If compassion is the hallmark of the New Zealand system, efficiency is the chief characteristic of the state-operated program for the blind in the Soviet Union. Anxious to learn more about the Soviet method of aiding the blind, I had written to officials in the field prior to my visit to Leningrad and Moscow in 1973. I never received a response from those rehabilitation officers, and I found making an appointment after my arrival in Moscow to be impossible.

I did learn that the Soviets follow a similar system employed in some of the eastern European nations. The government designates one factory to employ blind people and constructs apartment houses nearby to provide a "village" for all the visually handicapped. The system is one of almost total

198

segregation and while the Soviets regard the concept as efficient and humane, westerners tend to dislike the program because of the lack of individual choice.

Throughout my travels I have generally found that the places that utilize the most modern concepts of educating and rehabilitating the blind tend to be areas that once had a strong British influence. For example, the Hong Kong Society for the Blind operates a rehabilitation center and a factory primarily with blind employees that stresses giving the visually handicapped dignity through independence. I discovered a similar situation in India, where despite the overwhelming poverty of the nation as a whole, the programs for the blind in the urban areas seem relatively enlightened.

Over the past two decades by attending International Lions Conventions and meetings of global organizations for the blind, I have had the privilege of visiting many nations ranging from Israel, Egypt and Jordan to Japan, Taiwan and the People's Republic of China. In Wiesbaden, Germany I had a wonderful personal experience when I discovered the jewelry shop of my ancestor named Christoph Kumpe which dated back to 1810. As a part of that same trip we explored the Old Hesse area, including the lovely gardens that surround some of the local castles. On that particular occasion I felt a great sense of generational unity with my great-grandfather who, before journeying to America, began life as a gardener at one of those same castles.

No matter where we've traveled, I've observed that any place with a core of dedicated people who honestly believe in the ability and potential of the blind, is making progress toward creating a new life for the visually handicapped. While the world capitals I have been fortunate to visit are geographically a long way from Little Rock, I've always felt at home each time I've encountered those individuals, no matter what their nationality, who share my interest in the international rehabilitation movement.

Every career offers certain remunerations and I regard the friends I have made both here and abroad who have shared my zeal for our cause to be among the most rewarding aspect of my forty years in the work for the blind. A great sense of mission permeates our professional conferences and conventions which almost always seem like a reunion of old friends.

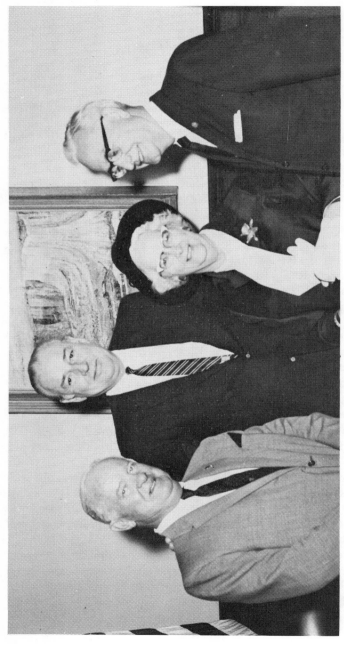

International trainees often had the opportunity to visit with government and business leaders. Kumpe and James S. Binder of Little Rock (left), then president of AEB, accompanied Mrs. Cecilia Savignac of Mexico City to visit Governor Winthrop Rockefeller in 1968.

Through the years I have attended hundreds of these meetings and each time I have found inspiration from the exchanges of ideas that mark the conferences and from the renewed sense of community that binds all of us together.

For many years I especially looked forward to certain national meetings because I knew I would have an opportunity to visit with Father Tom Carroll. Although Father Carroll was sighted, many people referred to him as the "Blind Priest" because of his dedication to helping the visually handicapped. I first encountered Father Carroll and his dynamic personality at a 1954 AAWB conference in Houston, Texas. That same year he founded the St. Paul's Rehabilitation Center in Newton, Massachusetts and from that time on, because of our mutual concerns and paralleled careers we became close friends.

Our relationship was often marked by friendly disagreements over how rehabilitation centers should be operated. Well into the 1960s Father Carroll and I continued to argue over his concept of rehabilitation as a group undertaking. He contended that the most efficient way of aiding the adult blind was to start a group of twelve or fourteen blind persons as a class and have them move through the various training disciplines together, participate in group therapy sessions and thereby eliminate the tremendous sense of loneliness that characterizes many recently blinded individuals.

I countered that no two people were alike and that from my own experience no pair of trainees progressed through their training at the same rate. Therefore, I argued a rehabilitation center should be based on a system of individualized instruction that recognized that all blind people are not the same. Although Father Carroll and I differed on other matters such as his proposal for separate training programs for the partially sighted, inspite of our friendly disagreements, we developed a bond of respect and admiration based on our shared goal of helping the blind.

Father Carroll served as the chaplain for the blinded veterans at the Old Farms Convalescent Hospital at Avon and also wrote a wonderful book entitled *Blindness: What It Is, What It Does, and How to Live With It,* which remains one of the best introductory works on the subject. I always had the greatest regard for Father Carroll and after the completion of the

AEB's new buildings, I invited him to participate in one of our training seminars in Little Rock.

During a tour of the facility, Father Carroll paused in front of the door to our techniques of daily living room. For some reason we had changed the terminology to daily demands of living and the sign on the door had been abbreviated to "Daily Demands." Father Carroll pointed at the sign and said, "Roy, is that the toilet?"

I always learned a lot from Father Carroll, even regarding small matters. Soon after his departure we returned to the term "techniques" of daily living and I quietly had the sign on the door changed.

Father Carroll's death in 1971 marked the passing of one of the dominant figures in the rehabilitation movement for an entire generation. A year later the directors of his center in Massachusetts appropriately renamed the facility the Carroll Rehabilitation Center for the Visually Impaired. Despite our philosophical differences, I regarded Father Carroll as one of the brightest and most dedicated members of our profession and I believe his numerous achievements are best measured by the thousands of blind people whose lives were enriched by the work of the "Blind Priest."

A second inspiring individual I met through my career in working with the visually handicapped was Dr. Richard Kinney. Blinded as a child, during his freshman year in college Dick also lost his hearing. In spite of his double handicap, he graduated summa cum laude from Mt. Union College in Ohio. He also took some correspondence courses from the Hadley School for the Blind in Winnetka, Illinois and so impressed the faculty there that they offered him a position at the institution.

Dick had a little more modulation in his voice than many deaf-blind individuals because he had once been able to hear and he became involved in the public relations activities of the school. He also married a blind girl, but she died suddenly, leaving Dick to raise their six-year-old son alone. With the assistance of his family, Dick reared the child himself while advancing over the years to the position of president of Hadley School.

Even though arthritis restricted him to a wheelchair later in his life, Dick traveled all over the world to promote the interests of the Hadley School and the education of the blind. He visited Little Rock on several occasions and in the mid-1970s I invited him to speak to one of our International Services for the Blind board meetings. During the course of Dick's stay in the city, Governor David Pryor commissioned him an "Arkansas Traveler," a state distinction presented to visiting dignitaries.

Before his death a couple of years ago, Dick wrote several moving poems about the nature of human existence for publication. In my estimation Richard Kinney was a great man whose dedication to life and service, despite his many handicaps, personified the concept of human courage.

A bold spirit also marked the career of Louis Rives, one of my closest friends in the rehabilitation movement. Blinded as an infant, Louis attended public schools in Virginia and later received both a bachelor's and a law degree from William and Mary College in Williamsburg. He began a distinguished career as a federal employee in 1943 when he joined the staff of the general counsel of the Federal Services Administration. I first met Lou while attending a training seminar in Washington, D. C. where he delivered an outstanding address explaining the implications of the new Barden-LaFollette legislation.

We became close friends after Lou became an assistant to the regional representative of the vocational rehabilitation office in Dallas. He visited our center in Little Rock on several occasions and he and I spent many hours discussing the future of the rehabilitation program. Eventually, Lou became the Chief of the Office of the Blind in Washington. In that capacity he supported the efforts of the AEB to acquire available grants, including the Hill-Burton funds for our first expansion program.

Lou later headed the Civil Rights Division of the Department of Social Rehabilitation Services, but at the age of fifty-five after thirty years as a federal employee he decided to retire. I happened to be in Washington when he announced his retirement, so I asked him if he planned to leave Washington. He told me he had considered several different places, but had not made a final decision. By coincidence I needed someone to direct our research grant program and so I suggested Lou consider retiring to Arkansas.

A few weeks later Lou and his wife, Marcy, came to Little Rock as our house guests to see what they thought of Arkansas and before they left, they made a down payment on a home in the city. Following his retirement Lou joined the AEB as the director of Research and Staff Development. During his tenure with us Lou also served as the president of the National Accreditation Council and with his knowledge of federal programs and his many friends in Washington, he secured several important grants for the center, including the initial funds that established the master's program at UALR.

In 1975, after a year and a half with the AEB, Lou received an appointment as the Administrator of the state Office for the Blind and Visually Impaired. Although I hated to lose such a valuable staff member, I felt the move would be to the advantage of all the blind people of Arkansas, and I especially wanted Lou to take the position since he would be the first blind person to head the agency.

Louis Rives did an excellent job in his new position as Administrator. After five years, however, he retired again, this time to the sunshine of Arizona. Like the telephone company television commercials, he and I still talk to each other over the phone about every two weeks. Lou's career had a great influence on the work for the blind throughout the nation and especially in Arkansas and I feel fortunate to have been a close friend of such a major figure in the rehabilitation movement.

Over the years I worked closely with many individuals who had a tremendous impact on the work for the blind - people like Robert Barnett, a bright young man from Florida who became the executive director of the American Foundation for the Blind at the age of thirty-one; Mary Switzer, a pioneer in the field who served as the head of the rehabilitation program in the Department of Health, Education and Welfare; and William Gallaher, the protege of Father Carroll who rose through the ranks to become the present executive director of the AFB. I feel privileged to have had the opportunity to experience a close relationship with dedicated individuals like these and many others. To have shared a sense of purpose with such outstanding people has been a never-ending source of inspiration for my own career.

In 1978 my commitment to aiding the visually handicapped entered a new phase with my retirement as the executive director of the AEB rehabilitation center in Little Rock. For a brief period my friend Howard H. Hanson, a former head of the state agency for the blind in South Dakota, directed the activities of the center until poor health forced him to relinquish the position. He was succeeded by Jim Cordell, a former teacher and basketball coach who joined our staff as a mobility instructor in 1961 and later served as my assistant executive director. Jim received a master's degree in orientation and mobility from Western Michigan University and married a charming former trainee named Elizabeth Young in the years before he assumed the directorship. Despite our policy against instructors dating students, I'll have to confess in the case of Jim and Beth, I tended to look the other way.

Over the past few years I have tried to maintain an active retirement by delivering numerous speeches and doing whatever I could to promote the cause of the rehabilitation of the blind. The AEB board designated me Founder Chairman Emeritus and combined with being president of the International Services for the blind, I have retained a busy involvement in the field.

One activity I have particularly enjoyed since I retired involved planning the Helen Keller Centennial Congress. Under the leadership of William Gallagher, the American Foundation for the Blind sponsored the event on June 27, 1980 in honor of the hundredth anniversary of Miss Keller's birth. Since Miss Keller attended both the Perkins School and Radcliffe College, we decided to hold the Congress in Boston. In planning the meeting we hoped to unite all the agencies and organizations of and for the blind to meet together for the first time and honor the remarkable Helen Keller.

Our committee started eighteen months in advance and we invited a galaxy of national and international figures to participate in the program. Kim Wickes, my friend from West Memphis, sang both the invocation and the benediction at the Congress and in between we held a series of seminars centering on the various phases of Helen Keller's career (Early Years, Working Years, Later Years). Arkansas was well represented since three of the four main seminars were chaired by people with ties to the state. I presided over the session covering Miss Keller's later years; Max Woolly, the superintendent of the Arkansas School for the Blind, conducted the meeting on the Early Years; and Lou Rives led the

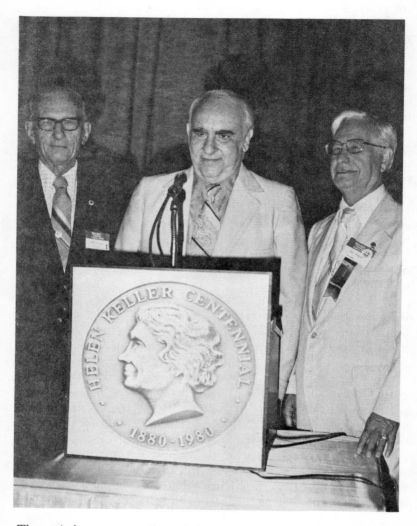

*Three Arkansans — (from left) J. M. Woolly, then superinten-
dent of the Arkansas School for the Blind; Louis Rives, Jr., then
administrator of the Arkansas State Office for the Blind and
Visually Impaired; and Roy Kumpe — were on the planning
committee and chaired three of the four seminars at the Helen
Keller Centennial in Boston, 1980.*

session entitled "The Rights and Responsibilities of the Blind."

During the seminars we used Helen Keller's life as a vehicle to review the entire history of the work for the blind, assess our efforts at the present time and speculate on the future direction of the movement. Along with the main seminars each organization held individual meetings and various groups sponsored exhibits throughout the course of the Congress.

By the time the meetings ended we all felt the event had succeeded in every way. The various gatherings were attended by over 2,700 people and the whole affair represented one of the rare high points of cooperation among the many groups involved in the education and rehabilitation of the blind. All organizations of and for the blind were represented, including the NFB, who picketed the National Accreditation Council's board meeting.

Along with professional commitments like the Helen Keller Congress, my retirement has been filled with activities that have been of lifelong interest. For example, since the days when I received my baptism in a creek and taught a Sunday School class at the age of sixteen, I have been interested in comparative religions. During my retirement I have found the time to study the great faiths of the world — Islam, Judaism, Buddhism, Hinduism and Christianity.

This inquiry has been more than just an intellectual amusement. One of the most disturbing characteristics of newly blinded adults is a tendency to suffer severe religious crises. Often our trainees questioned their own faith and many blamed God for their plight. Several even raised provocative questions regarding the nature of a kind and merciful God who had suddenly made them blind. Others became despondent waiting for a religious miracle to restore their lost sight. Having experienced a close relationship with so many individuals who felt victimized by their own god, I have found the study of religions to be of more value than a simple academic exercise.

On the other hand, my personal religious activities have been an endless source of strength and inspiration over the years. After marrying Berenice I joined the Christian Church and as I often tell my friends "I was reared a Baptist, married a Campbellite and she made a Christian out of me." Following

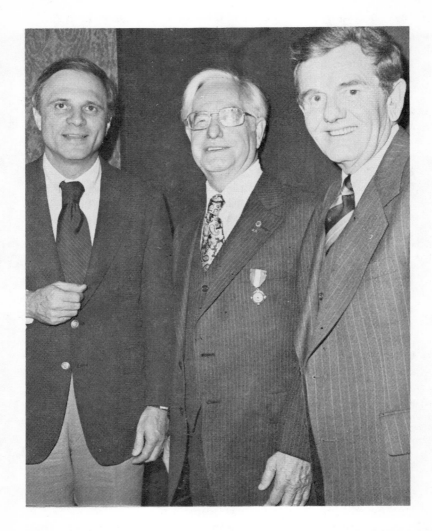

Two of the speakers at Roy Kumpe's 1978 retirement dinner in Little Rock's Camelot Inn were (left) Governor (now U. S. Senator) David Pryor and (right) Joseph M. McLoughlin of South Norwalk, Conn., the 61st president of Lions International. Kumpe wears the personal medal President McLoughlin presented to him that evening.

the Second World War, Berenice and I helped found the "Friendly Class," a Sunday school class for young couples. Our group has stayed together and the "Friendly Class" still plays an active role in our church and in our lives. I have always believed in serving God through serving mankind and have tried to structure my life on that premise not only in my professional life but also in serving as a Sunday school teacher for a term and as an elder and chairman of our church board.

Another area of service that has highlighted my retirement involves the realization of a fifty-two year old dream. During my senior year at the Arkansas School for the Blind a good friend and fellow student approached me one day and said, "Roy, if you graduate from here and then go to college and study law, someday you could come back and be the superintendent of the school for the blind."

I laughed and said, "Heck, I don't want to be the superintendent. I want to be on the board and hire the superintendent!"

In January, 1981 Governor Frank White appointed me to the Board of Trustees of the Arkansas School for the Blind, fulfilling my dream of over half a century. After 43 years as principal and superintendent, Dr. J. Max Woolly retired, and I realized my ambition by participating in the selection of Dr. Hugh Pace as superintendent, thus enabling me to make a contribution to the institution where I began my career.

Of course, another part of my community service has centered on my work with Lions Clubs. Entering my forty-second year as a Lions Club member, I have attended forty state conventions and seventeen international conventions. In 1958 I helped organize the Park Plaza Lions Club in suburban Little Rock and served as first president. A few years later I served a term as a Lions District Governor.

One Lions function I have particularly enjoyed over the years is the annual Visiting District Governors' Day under the sponsorship of the Arkansas Lions and the AEB. Back in 1961, with my encouragement Ed Barry took the initiative of inviting the District Governors from Arkansas' six adjoining states to come to Little Rock and see our rehabilitation center firsthand. Initially we hoped this event would publicize the center and provide an understanding of our training of the blind who came to AEB from their states. In the last few years, however, under the leadership of Dr. Jim Fowler the event has grown to have international significance in the Lions movement. As a member of the board of Lions International, Jim began inviting all the international officers and board members to Little Rock for the District Governors' Day. Eventually we added an International Family Night and by the early 1980s the Visiting District Governors' Day has become one of the largest meetings of Lions dignitaries in the United States. Another welcomed result of this meeting is the fact that many other states have adopted AEB as their Lions Clubs' project and support it financially.

The Lions Club has been an integral part of my life for almost half a century. The group has provided me with a vehicle for service and a social outlet and, although I recognize businessmen's luncheon clubs are not without their critics, the Lions Club has been a positive factor in my life for over four decades.

Participation in the Lions Club and the church combined with various professional commitments have made retirement a lively period in my life. I have slowed down to some extent, which has given me the opportunity to reflect upon the events, activities and rewards of the past half century.

Part of my reflections have quite naturally centered on my visual handicap. While I believe dwelling on what-might-have-been to be a pointless exercise, nevertheless, my lack of sight has unquestionably had an impact on the direction of my life. There have been occasions when I believed that other people, upon discovering my handicap suddenly felt I lacked the competence of a fully sighted person. Many times whether in politics or business or in my work at the AEB, I experienced this subtle form of discrimination. Consequently, I think one of my underlying goals throughout my career has been to hasten the day when we will all judge people by their abilities and not their disabilities.

Adjusting to partial sight has also been characterized by inconvenience and a few embarrassing moments. Probably the most awkward incident in this regard took place at a new eating establishment in North Little Rock some years ago. We were dining with the chairman of the AEB board and as we left the restaurant I moved ahead of our party to admire the decorative statues in the foyer of the building. I reached out and touched one of the figures as I had done with the cathedral sculptures in Europe. When I realized I was touching real flesh I immediately said "Excuse me." Just then our board chairman arrived and I told him I thought the woman was a statue.

He quickly turned to the lady and said, "You'll have to excuse him, he's blind, and he thought you were a statue."

The woman proceeded to rescue me to some extent by replying, "Oh well. That's all right. I *am* stoned."

Throughout my childhood in rural Pulaski County, our roads were unpaved and inevitably, following a heavy rain, at least one automobile would become stuck in the mud somewhere near Ironton. On most of these occasions my father would hitch his team of mules to the wagon and ride off to offer his assistance to the stranded motorists. I enjoyed riding to the rescue with him although he always puzzled me by refusing to accept any rewards from the grateful individuals whose cars had been pulled from the muck. My father always politely refused the offers of money saying, "All you owe me is to help the next guy you find stuck in the mud."

From my father's example I developed a philosophy of service and as I grew older the idea of helping others became the cornerstone of my career. Even though I did find a measure of happiness and success in politics and business, my primary concern has always been aiding the blind.

Blindness remains no respector of persons and no one has been able to eradicate the fact that human beings do lose their sight. But in the brief span of my own career the quality of blind people's existence has been greatly improved. Although much remains to be done, in the last half century a virtual revolution has taken place in terms of the possibilities for the visually handicapped. Many factors have influenced this revolution, including new vocational opportunites, aided by enlightened attitudes on the part of many employers and corporations; increased chances for blind people to acquire college educations; positive legislation assisting those with visual handicaps, especially Section 504 of the Rehabilitation Act of 1973 (sometimes called the Civil Rights for the Handicapped Act because it prohibits discrimination against the handicapped); a new public awareness of the capabilities of the blind; and radical new technologies like the Optacon and Kurzweil Reader.

I believe the Arkansas Enterprises for the Blind has also played a part in improving the lives of blind people. By June of 1982 the center we opened in the Brack Home in 1947 with two trainees had served over 5,000 individuals from fifty states and fifty-three other countries. Our physical plant had expanded from a single rented residence to a facility valued at over three million dollars. As a result of the close cooperation between the state agencies serving the blind, the federal government and the Lions Clubs of Arkansas, we fashioned a new approach to increase the opportunities for the adult blind to create a new life for themselves. Because a few dedicated men believed that blind people could become useful and productive citizens dependent on themselves and not on charity, we were able to create an institution that housed numerous, often unnoticed stories of courage and determination.

Somewhere in the 1980s, an eight-year-old boy will suffer the loss of sight much as I did over sixty years ago and I'm sure he will undergo the same traumatic adjustments I experienced. Hopefully though, if we have done our work well, his opportunites of fulfilling his own potential and creating a meaningful life have increased a hundredfold over those sixty years. If that is the case then my own journey will have been a successful one.

Appendix

Editor's Note: Mr. Kumpe's awards include the following honors:

Migel Medal — American Foundation for the Blind

Shotwell Award — American Association of Workers for the Blind

Founders Award — *Dialogue* (a nationally produced magazine for the blind)

Meritorious Service Award — Southwest Region of the National Rehabilitation Association

Ambassador Award — American Council of the Blind

Distinguished Service Award — National Association of Rehabilitation Facilities

Marion Mill Preminger Medallion — People-to-People Committee for the Handicapped

Lions International Ambassador of Goodwill and Humanitarian Award

Little Rock Junior College Alumnus of the Year Award

"Boss of the Year" — Little Rock Jaycees

"Little Rockian of the Year" — readers of the *Arkansas Democrat*

Honorary Doctorate of Law Degree — University of Arkansas at Fayetteville

Bibliographical Essay

The best starting place for any reader interested in the modern history of the blind in America is Frances A. Koestler, *The Unseen Minority: A Social History of Blindness in the United States* (New York: David McKay Company, Inc., 1976). The book is an indispensable and well-written introduction to the organizations and personalities that have shaped the course of the movement to aid the visually handicapped in the twentieth century.

On the nature of blindness, I would highly recommend Reverend Thomas J. Carroll, *Blindness, What It Is, What It Does, and How To Live With It* (Boston: Little Brown and Co., 1961). Father Carroll's analysis of the many implications of blindness has been unsurpassed for over twenty years.

For the behind-the-scenes story of the passage of the Randolph-Sheppard Act see Leonard A. Robinson, *Light at the Tunnel End* (Silver Springs, Maryland: Foundation for the Handicapped and Elderly, Inc., 1975). Regarding additional specific topics, Kenneth L. Jernigan and the National Federation of the Blind receive a lengthy and relatively balanced treatment in Carl Bakal, *Charities, USA* (New York: New York Times Book Company, 1979).

I would also suggest Lucy Ching, *One of the Lucky Ones* (Hong Kong: Gulliver Books, 1980), which is one of the most moving accounts of a single individual's struggle with blindness that I have ever encountered. Of course, another excellent first-hand work is the Helen Keller classic, *The Story of My Life* (New York: Doubleday Doran, 1939). A more recent and highly readable volume on Miss Keller's life and work is Joseph P. Lash, *Helen and Teacher: The Story of Helen Keller and Anne Sullivan Macy* (New York: Delacorte Press, 1980), a

214

detailed but absorbing story of courage and determination based upon the most modern scholarly investigations.

Serious students of the subject of blindness should also consult the numerous publications of the American Association of Workers for the Blind and the American Foundation for the Blind.

The spirit of Lions International is captured in Julien Hyer, *Texas Lions, 1917-67* (Waco: Hill Junior College Press, 1969). The book also contains a brief history of the early years of the national Lions Club movement.

The main source for additional material on the Arkansas Enterprises for the Blind is the AEB's monthly newsletter, *New Life*. Back issues of *New Life* from 1954 are contained in a set of bound volumes at the rehabilitation center. The files of the *Arkansas Gazette* and the *Arkansas Democrat* also contain news articles from the AEB's inception in 1939 to the present.

INDEX

218

Lions Clubs of Arkansas, 57-60, 62, 82, 83, 95, 103, 109, 125, 130, 131, 133, 135, 150, 151, 183, 191, 192, 209, 210, 212.
Lions Club Park Plaza, 209.
Lions Club of Pine Bluff, 97.
Lions Club of Nashville, Arkansas, 100.
Lions Club of England, Arkansas, 122.
Lions Club - Pulaski Heights, 127.
Lions Club - Pine Bluff Evening, 148.
Ludden, Richard, 116.

—M—

MacFarland, Douglas, 122, 138.
Magers, George, 138.
Matilda Ziegler Magazine for the Blind, 25.
McCahill, William, 79.
McCullough, Robert, 118.
McDaniel, Ann, 142, 143.
McDaniels, Durwood, 186.
McLoughlin, Joseph M., 1, 208.
McSpadden, Jack, 139.
Metcalfe, Rena, 115.
Meyers, Charles, 48.
Miller, Betty, 112, 113.
Mills, Wilbur, 70, 124.
Minneapolis Society for the Blind, 173, 174.
Murphy, J.O., 138.
Mussa, Matthew, 197.

—N—

Nash, William, 182.
National Accreditation Council for Agencies Serving the Blind (N.A.C.), 157, 158, 172-74, 183, 184, 186, 204, 207.
National Federation of the Blind, 170-86.
New Zealand Foundation for the Blind, 197, 198.
Norvell, Hugo, 41, 43, 52.

—O—

Odom, Jess, 95, 120, 121, 125, 127, 136.

Office for Blind and Visually Impaired of Arkansas, 135, 139, 204.
Office of Vocational Rehabilitation of Arkansas, 34, 44, 52, 157, 165, 167.
Optacon, 160, 161, 163, 165, 168, 212.

—P—

P.L. 94142 (Mainstreaming), 147.
Pace, Hugh, 209.
Pan-American Health Organization, 192.
Park, Yong Bong, 188-90.
Partners of the Americas, 192.
Penix, Ray, 178, 179.
Penman, Evelyn, 106.
Perkins School for the Blind, 160, 188, 205.
Peters, Dick, 162.
Pinkerton, Grace Noyes, 121-23, 127, 132, 136.
Pipkin, John, 61, 154.
Potter, Stanley, 164.
Pradilla, Hernando, 195-97.
President's Committee on Employment of the Handicapped, 79, 81, 82.
Price, Stanley, 124, 131.
Projects With Industry, 141.
Pryor, David, 1, 70, 126, 127, 203, 208.

—R—

Randolph, Jennings, 26.
Randolph-Sheppard Act, 25, 26, 60, 77, 79, 181, 186.
Reaves, Lee, 71.
Rehabilitation Act of 1973, 211.
Rehabilitation Service Administration (U.S.), 145.
Riedel, Candy, 104, 105, 107, 127.
Riley, Bob, 69, 70.
Rives, Louis, 98, 167, 185, 203-06.
Robinson, Leonard A., 25, 139, 186.
Rockefeller, Winthrop, 70, 129, 200.
Roose, Sylvia, 109, 110.
Ross, Ashley, 24, 52, 60-62, 135.